EAT YOURSELF
THIN
FAT BITCH

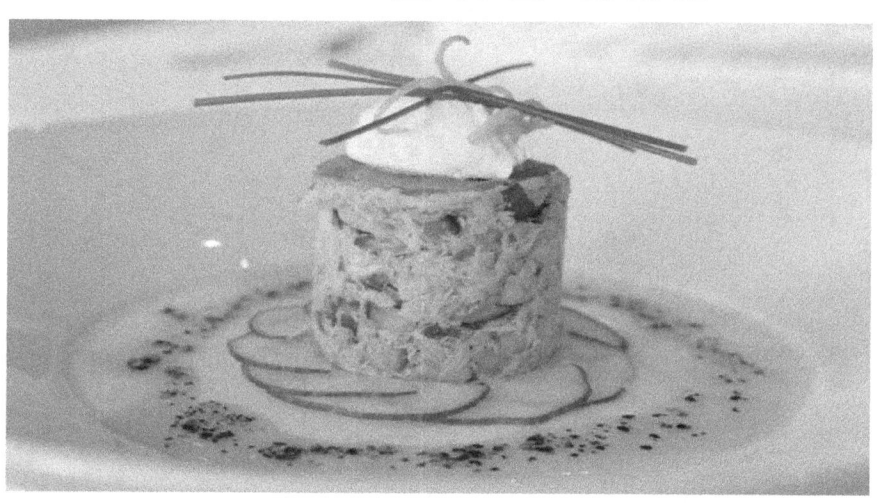

20 SCIENTIFICALLY PROVEN WAYS TO
LOSE WEIGHT AND BURN FAT

DAVID E. MALOCCO

B.Sc., B.C.L., Dip. F.Sc., Dip. P.C.P.

ISBN: **1530037670**
ISBN-13: **978-1530037674**

DEDICATION

To Colette, for her patience.

CONTENTS

ACKNOWLEDGMENTS

The author would like to thank Gary Power for his design and cover and also the following: Dr. Spencer Nadolsky, J.J. Virgin, Dr. Amy Shah, Dr. Jane Teas, Jennifer Di Noia, Dr. Oz, Dr. Jeremy Burton, and Dr. Didier Raoult.

The author would also like to thank the following bodies: National Cancer Institute, University of Carolina, Harvard University, Texas Woman's University, William Patterson University, Rochester Center for Obesity, America Food Standards Agency, American Society for Clinical Nutrition, Canadian Research and Development Centre for Probiotics, American H Association Advisory and Co-Ordinating Committee, and the Specialty Food Association of America.

Finally, the author would like to thank the following publications: Biology Letters, Journal of Lipid Research, Journal of Food Science, International Journal of Obesity, Journal of Clinical Psychiatry, British Journal of Nutrition, British Medical Journal, and the Journal of Nutrition.

1 WHY BUY THIS BOOK

First of all, don't blame yourself because you are overweight. Instead, congratulate yourself for doing something about it and buying this book. There may be several reasons why you are overweight and none of them may have anything to do with gluttony. So, don't fall into the trap of beating yourself up.

The fact is that now, you accept, that like most of us, you need to lose some weight. You want to look better, be healthier and feel happier. But, you don't know where to start. There is so much contradictory advice out there. Eat this, don't eat this. Do this, don't do this. For this reason I decided to write a simple, straightforward book about how to lose and control your weight using scientifically proven evidence.

In other words, when I advise you to eat something or not eat something, I will produce the scientific evidence to back up this advice. It will not be just my opinion it will be my opinion supported by documented scientific evidence that what I am telling you actually works.

To lose weight is not simply a question of dieting. It's more of a change of lifestyle. That is not to say dieting does not work. It can work and I have given you the world's four most successful diets at the end of this book with sample daily menus if that's the route you want to take. But, before you have the urge to skip to those pages now allow me to explain a thing or two about what is actually involved in losing weight.

In order to lose and control weight effectively you need to know five things:

- What to eat
- What not to eat
- What to drink
- How to exercise, and
- Some essential medical advice.

Also, it is important to remember that different foods work better for different people. Therefore, different diets work better for different people. No one diet fits everyone. That's why many diets will work for some but not others. This book will help you lose weight. It will tell you what food to eat – foods that work for everyone. It will explain why there are particular types of food you should never eat.

I will also reveal the ten most common weight loss mistakes that people make – usually on the advice of unprofessional nutritionists. I will explain to you what exactly protein and carbs mean; why eating a "low fat" diet can be absolutely useless for certain people; why you should always avoid fruit juices; why thinking that you need to eat three substantial meals a day is idiotic; the importance of eggs (including yolks) in your daily diet; how all calories are not created equally, and why you need to stop believing what the media writes about weight loss.

If you follow the basic twenty rules that I give you in this book then you will lose weight and you will be able to control your weight. That's a fact. Guaranteed. Proven. Given. You can create your own diet and often that's a better way because it makes it much easier for you. No one wants to have to eat food they don't like. And the fact is, you don't have to. Even if you comply 60-75% with my rules you will lose weight. Don't worry if it doesn't happen immediately. The chances are it will take you at least two weeks to see a drop in your weight. In that time, you might actually feel and look worse. Why?

Because your body and mind is adjusting to change and trying how best to cope with that change. This is a good thing. Losing weight should be fun. If it's not fun, then you're doing something wrong. As well as changing the food you eat you need to take certain exercise. I will tell you the type of exercises you can take. They don't have to be rigorous exercises, not at all. Everything in this book is designed to help you lose weight with the minimum amount of effort. You can do it. You will do it. Follow the rules I give you and trust me you will thank me for it.

So, what's keeping you? Let's get started.

PART 1

2 WHAT TO EAT

RULE #1. ADD PROTEIN TO YOUR DIET

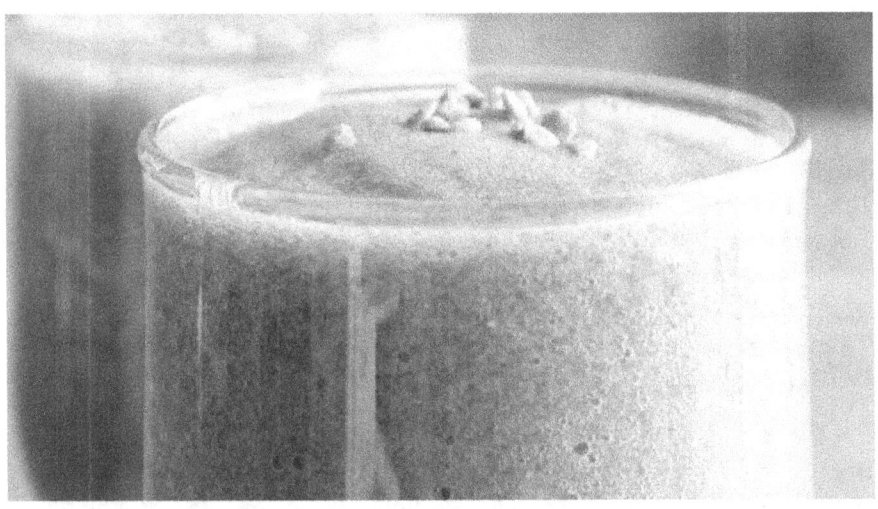

Adding protein to your daily diet is the easiest, most effective and delicious way to lose weight with the least amount of effort. In fact, if you were to follow just one of the twenty rules in this book this is by far the most important.

According to Americas' nutrition expert, Dr. Spencer Nadolsky "Protein is King." Why? I hear you ask. Eating protein is one of the fastest ways to calm your hunger and sugar cravings. You probably knew that protein is great for keeping you satisfied, but did you know it can also decrease your cravings? How so? Because protein slows down our neuronal reward system.

The neuronal reward system relates to the chemicals in the brain that make us feel good and motivate us to eat more food, even during those times when we're not hungry. When we're low in protein, our food cravings take over, looking for a quick fix. In one scientific study, 25% of calories as protein reduced obsessive thoughts about food by 60%. It also reduced the desire for the late-night snacking curse by 50%.

If your goal is to lose and control your weight, with minimal effort, then you should definitely increase your protein intake. Not only will it help you lose weight, it will also prevent or at least significantly reduce weight regain.

A huge amount of studies prove that protein both increases your metabolic rate and helps reduce appetite. Protein requires energy to metabolize, accordingly, a high protein diet can increase calories burned by up to 80 to 100 calories per day. Not only that, but protein is also the most fulfilling nutrient, by far. One study proved that those who consumed 30% of calories as protein automatically ate 441 fewer calories every day.

What this means is that it is easily possible to increase calories output and reduce calories intake simply by adding protein to your diet. This is the most important weight loss factor there is. If the only thing you change as a result of reading this book is to permanently increase your protein intake, then you will be well on your way towards lowering your weight, maintaining that decrease and working towards a healthier body in the long-term.

The fact is that when you get a sudden craving for sugar, your body is really crying out for protein. When you are low in protein, your system knows it needs energy. Because you need energy, you crave foods that will give you fuel fast. These are usually high-sugar impact foods that you're in the mood for.

Unfortunately, these are precisely the type of foods that will raise your blood sugar and trigger an insulin response. This then shuts off fat burning. What can you do? Well instead of eating a cookie, try eating a handful of almonds or a low-fat plain Greek yogurt. In that way, you'll curb cravings for sweets by giving your body the kind of sustained energy it really needs.

HOW MUCH PROTEIN?

How much protein should you consume each day? One study concluded that 25 - 30 grams of protein at each meal will benefit weight loss, appetite and other health factors. Experts suggest that the average woman should consume 75 - 80 grams daily, whereas most men should consume 100 - 120 grams of protein a day. That equates to roughly four to six ounces for women or six to eight ounces for men for each meal. These numbers can vary as obviously your existing weight and body composition will influence the amount of protein you need. Remember that those needs will increase if you're under stress, if you're healing or if you're engaged in heavy resistance training.

THE RIGHT PROTEIN

What is the right protein source for your diet? Experts agree that the best sources of protein include high-quality animal protein, including grass-fed beef, free-range chicken, wild-caught low-mercury fish and providing you are not intolerant, eggs. This can sometimes be difficult for vegans and vegetarians. But there are plenty of plant-based high-protein foods you can use like quinoa, legumes, nuts and seeds.

Breakfast is the best time to start your protein intake. Studies show that a high-protein breakfast suppresses ghrelin, your hunger hormone, far better than a high-carbohydrate breakfast. They also found that a moderate or high-protein breakfast curbed cravings in overweight and obese young people. So, rather than consuming a carbohydrate-rich breakfast like cereal that will leave you hungry a couple of hours later, why not try a protein shake? According to nutritionist J. J. Virgin her number one game changer for fast, lasting fat has nothing to do with exercise or changing what goes on to your plate. It's all to do with a protein shake.

A protein shake takes five minutes to prepare and provides all the nutrients you need to perform effectively. At the same time it keeps you full, focused, and burning fat for hours. Studies confirm a liquid meal replacement "can safely and effectively produce significant sustainable weight loss and improve weight-related risk factors of disease."

While a delicious muffin or "health conscious" cereal will instigate a blood sugar surge, creating hunger and cravings throughout the day, a protein shake steadies blood sugar levels to keep hunger and cravings at bay. It's a win win situation.

More than anything else, I recommend protein shakes to start your day off. Why? Because they are simple, particularly if you haven't got time to spend preparing your breakfast or need to get kids out the door. They also provide steady, sustained energy.

Let's say that at the moment your normal breakfast consists of a low-fat muffin and large latte. This type of breakfast is guaranteed to raise your insulin levels and increase your stress hormone cortisol. It will cause a late morning crash resulting in a crave for another sugary, caffeinated pick-me-up. But a protein shake will provide you with sustained energy until lunchtime.

Not only is is healthier but it is significantly more cost effective. If you don't eat breakfast at home calculate how much you spend on take-away coffees, smoothies, fruit juices, Danish, muffins etc. Each one of these will increase your weight. A protein shake, on the other hand, will fill you up, provide you with nutrients and burn fat. You don't buy a protein shake. You can. But don't. Make your own. I am going to give you a recipe that will provide you with an excellent source of healthy fat, fiber, antioxidants, and nutrients. All you need do is pour them into a blender, press the button and pour.

HOW TO MAKE A GREAT PROTEIN SHAKE
This is what you need:
A non-soy, non dairy plant-based or defatted-beef powder with 20 - 25 grams of protein and 5 grams or less of sugar per serving. (Readily available in any decent health shop).
½ cup - 1 cup frozen berries (strawberries, blackberries or raspberries work best)
A handful of Spinach, Kale or other leafy greens
1 - 2 Tbsp freshly ground flaxseed or chia seeds (Again, readily available from any health shop).
8 - 10 ounces unsweetened coconut or almond milk
One skinned and de-stoned Avocado
Swap this protein shake for your normal breakfast every morning for two weeks and see the difference.

HEALTH WARNING
WHAT TO AVOID IN YOUR SHAKE
But be careful. While you can improvise on the ingredients do not change it by turning it into a milk-shake. Do not add high-sugar ingredients like dried fruit, sweetened nut milks and sugar-added almond butter as this will transform your healthy shake into a sugar-loaded, fat-storing disaster.

Next, a word about choosing the wrong protein. Finding the right protein shake can be challenging. Whey is the second most abundant protein in milk after casein. But the problem with whey is that it absorbs very quickly. That might be fine following a workout, but as a breakfast meal replacement whey becomes a disaster. In fact, one study shows that whey creates an insulin-raising effect similar to white bread, which explains why you're hungry an hour after a whey shake.

Casein protein is another one to avoid like the plague. While it absorbs more slowly than whey, casein peptides behave very similarly to gluten in that they can react with opiate receptors in the brain, mimicking drug like effects.

Forget about soy. Really, I hear you say. Yes, really. Health expert, Dr. Amy Shah says soy can adversely affect your thyroid and potentially contribute to breast cancer. As well as that, most soy is genetically modified (GMO). The solution is to choose non-soy, non dairy protein powder. My favorite plant proteins include rice, pea, chia, chlorella or cranberry protein.

Another smart option is defatted beef protein powder which provides whey's creaminess without dairy's reactivity. But, whichever you choose, your powder should contain 20 — 25 grams of protein per serving. You can increase this intake to 30 grams or more if you're very athletic, have significant weight to lose, or recovering from surgery or injury.

Read all labels carefully and avoid buying powders with unhealthy ingredients. Some manufacturers make powders palatable with preservatives, maltodextrin, fructose and other sugars, excessive sugar alcohols, and artificial sweeteners. Don't touch them. Buy professional brands, and opt for protein powders with fewer ingredients that are low-sugar impact. Do not choose a product that has more than five grams of added sugar per 100-calorie serving, and of course less is even better.

Try my shake first and see how it works. Then when you see the benefits and know a little bit more try changing the products to suit your own taste buds.

RULE #2. EAT FRUIT AND VEGETABLES

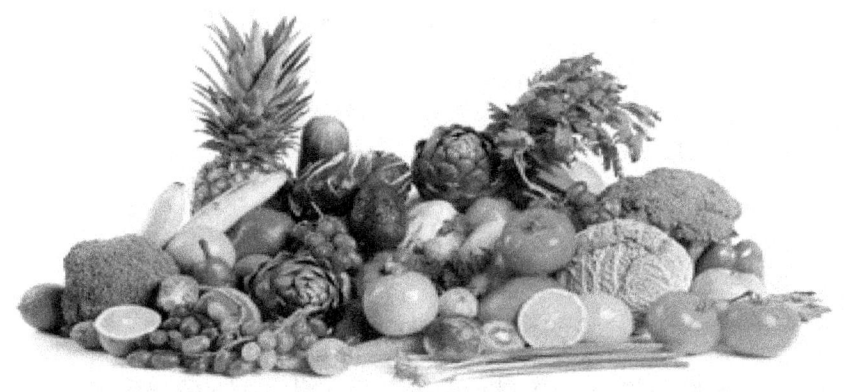

Let's talk about fruit first. Contrary to popular belief, not all fruit is created equal. There are certain fruits which are higher in fiber and pectin, both natural fat burners that can help you boost your metabolism. When eaten in excess some fruits contain high levels of natural sugar. However, other fruits, when consumed in the right amounts, actually help you to lose weight. Papaya, for instance, contains an enzyme called papain which promotes the faster transit of food through the stomach which can help to shed the pounds. So what I am saying is that not all fruits have the same nutritional value. I will tell you what fruits to eat.

The great thing about fruit is that it is perfect for snacking if you are trying to lose weight. The bad thing is that recently it has had some bad press in relation to its sugar content. But like most media reports these reports have been somewhat exaggerated.

Of course fruit does contain natural sugars but as you're eating it as a whole fruit, as opposed to a juice or smoothie, the fiber helps you absorb the sugars more slowly, making it more healthy. But the first important point to remember is to forget that "five a day" crap. Be careful to limit your portions of fruit to just two a day and watch the portion size.

If possible, try adding some protein to the fruit like nuts and seeds which will help slow down the absorption of sugars even more. If using dried fruit try soaking it in water first. This will fill you up more so you'll actually feel like eating less. By balancing your fruit with a protein and/or fat component you help stabilize your blood sugar levels. This is vital for weight loss.

If taking fruit as a mid-morning snack, always consider fruits which are rich in fiber. Pears and apples both have a high fiber content. Eating one medium sized apple or pear will help you feel fuller for longer, therefore aiding weight loss.

Media reports would have us believe that we should avoid fruit and vegetables like bananas, avocados, sweetcorn, peas and carrots because they are fattening. In contrast, they tell us to eat celery or grapefruit as these will actually help weight loss. But is this true?

Well, bananas, avocados, sweetcorn, peas and carrots are certainly higher in calories than most other fruit and vegetable. For example, you could eat two small apples for around the same amount of calories as a banana. Similarly, you could eat six times more spinach to provide you with the same amount of calories provided by sweetcorn. But while avocados are higher in fat than most other vegetables, most of this fat is heart-healthy monounsaturates, which comes in a package with plenty of vitamin E.

The good thing about avocado is that it has been shown to increase the metabolic rate as well as up testosterone production, the hormone responsible for weight loss in both men and women. So, despite the fact that these fruit and vegetables contain more calories, that doesn't mean you should avoid them. They are still an important source of many different nutrients. The key is to add them to your food diary so that the calories they provide are included in your daily total.

While foods like celery and grapefruit are certainly very low in calories, there's no conclusive evidence that eating them will actually help you burn off calories or make you lose weight. While some studies have shown that adding grapefruit to your diet will help shift those pounds, the jury is still out. And as for it taking more calories to digest a stick of celery than it actually provides, well, let's just say I'm not convinced.

HOW MUCH FRUIT AND VEG SHOULD YOU EAT?

That's a good question. Studies show that we tend to eat the same volume or weight of food every day, irrespective of its calorie content. So, if we want to lose weight, it's important, in fact, vital that you stick to lower calorie foods to make up this volume. And that's where fruit and vegetables play an important part in a weight loss diet. Many fruits and vegetables actually weigh a lot but they don't provide that many calories.

For example, a meal consisting of a 150g grilled chicken breast, a 300g jacket potato, 20g of butter and 30g low fat cheese provides a total weight of 500g and provides 790 calories. But if you substitute this meal for a 130g chicken breast, a 200g potato, 5g of butter, 80g broccoli, 45g carrots and 40g green salad, you still have an overall weight of 500g, but for just 480 calories. You will feel just as full after either meal but with the second choice you save 310 calories in a day which is the equivalent to half of one pound in a week and you haven't even changed the quantity of food you have eaten.

PORTION CONTROL

Remember, I told you never to eat more than two portions of fruit per day. One portion of fruit or vegetable is equivalent to 80g. Below are some examples of what counts as one portion:

1 apple, orange, pear or banana
3 heaped tablespoons of vegetables, beans or pulses
3 heaped tablespoons of fruit salad or stewed fruit
1 heaped tablespoon of raisins or sultanas
3 dried apricots
2 plums, satsumas, kiwi fruit or other similar sized fruit
1/2 a grapefruit or avocado
1 large slice of melon or fresh pineapple
1 cupful of grapes, cherries or berries
7 medium sized strawberries
1 small glass (150ml) of pure fruit juice
2 plums, satsumas, kiwi fruit or other similar sized fruit
1 dessert bowl of salad
1 large slice of melon or fresh pineapple

THE BEST FRUIT AND VEG TO EAT

MELONS
The watermelon is the number one fruit for weight loss. It's high in water content (90%) and a 100g serving just contains 30 calories. They're also a rich source of amino acids called arginine which helps burn fat. But probably the best thing about watermelon is that not only does it keep you hydrated, it will also keep you satiated for a long time which will lead to less unhealthy snacking.

Cantaloupes are extremely filling fruits and a cup of this type of melon, which contains only 60 calories, is enough to keep you full for a long time.

GUAVA
Introduced to India by Portuguese explorers the guava is packed with immense health benefits. It is high in fiber and is another potent weight loss aid due to the fact that its glycemic index is low. This makes it perfect for diabetics as well. Not only that but it keeps our bowel movements in excellent working order which helps the overall weight loss process.

APPLES
Believe it or not the humble apple is the one fruit that can reduce your cancer risk, keep your heart healthy, make your teeth whiter, boost your immune system and even beat diarrhea and constipation. If you're trying to lose weight then an apple a day is crucial to that plan. One medium-sized apple contains around 50 calories and doesn't have any fat or sodium. In fact, a Brazilian study found that women who ate apples before their meals lost 33% more calories than those who didn't eat them!

BANANAS
Number four on my list is the banana. Have a banana! Packing 100 calories, per piece, the average banana is an excellent source of instant energy and the perfect post-workout food. They are also healthier than packaged post-workout snacks like energy bars which are just chocolate bars pretending to be 'healthy' food bars. Bananas also aid muscle cramps, keep your blood pressure in check, prevent acidity and even beat constipation. High in both fiber and potassium they are an excellent weight loss fruit.

PEARS
A pear fulfils one quarter of your daily fiber requirement and is great for your digestive system. It also helps reduce cholesterol levels, reduces the risk of coronary heart diseases and type II diabetes and is rich in Vitamin C.

ORANGES

Not only do they taste great but 100g of this fruit contains a measly 47 calories which makes it perfect for that mid-day snack. Orange is a really great metabolism booster which is high in vitamin C, thiamin and folate. But don't make the fatal mistake of substituting orange juice for real oranges. This is a definite no-no. Oranges contain a lot less calories than orange juice and a lot less sugar. Also, they provide you with fiber which is not present in its juice form. In fact, you would be wise to leave orange juice out of your diet altogether.

TOMATOES

Tomatoes are packed with Vitamin C and lycopene. Lycopene stimulates the production of carnitine which is an amino acid that accelerates the body's fat burning process. They are full of antioxidants and reduce water retention. But remember tomatoes are tomatoes, ketchup is not tomatoes. Don't ever substitute ketchup for tomatoes.

In addition to their vibrancy and flavor, tomatoes, and in particular, organic tomatoes, are packed with nutrition, including a variety of phytochemicals that boast a long list of health benefits.

Tomatoes are an excellent source of lutein, zeaxanthin, and vitamin C (which is most concentrated in the jelly-like substance that surrounds the seeds), as well as vitamins A, E, and the B vitamins, potassium, manganese, and phosphorus.

Tomatoes are also a particularly concentrated source of lycopene. This is a carotenoid antioxidant that provides fruit and vegetables like tomatoes and watermelon a pink or red color. Lycopene's antioxidant activity has long been suggested to be more powerful than other carotenoids such as beta-carotene. In fact, scientific research suggests it may significantly lower your risk for stroke and cancer.

It's estimated that 85 percent of dietary lycopene in North Americans comes from tomato products such as tomato juice or tomato paste. In addition to lowering your risk for stroke, lycopene from tomatoes has also been deemed helpful in treating prostate cancer.

If you must consume ketchup, choose organic ketchup as it's been found to contain 57 percent more lycopene than conventional national brands. You should always store your tomatoes at room temperature; ideally, only store them in glass to reduce your BPA and phthalate exposure.

It would also be wise to cook any canned or bottled tomatoes as they tend to accumulate methanol very similar to aspartame. However, if you heat the tomatoes, the methanol is highly volatile and will boil away.

BLUEBERRIES
Blueberries are considered by many as the wonder fruit. They certainly are special and contain one of the highest antioxidant levels. They combat the factors that result in metabolic syndrome. This means that blueberries tackle insulin resistance, hypertension, obesity, and cholesterol. One study at the Texas Women's University (TWU) proved that blueberries fight fat cells. They are probably the best berry you can eat.

STRAWBERRIES
Strawberries are also a great weight loss fruit because they promote the production of the hormones adiponectin and leptin. Both of these are fat-burning hormones and metabolic boosters. This results in a higher metabolism when eaten in portion control along with a healthy, well balanced diet. They also have anti-inflammatory enzymes, which can help heal internal injuries or even tissue damage.

Berries contain concentrated amounts of the disease-fighting phytochemicals found to boost your immunity, prevent cancer, protect your heart, and prevent seasonal allergies. Berries are lower in sugar than many fruits, so they are less likely to destabilize your insulin levels.

Women who eat more than three servings of blueberries and strawberries per week have been found to enjoy a 32 percent lower risk of heart attack, due to the fruits' high anthocyanin content. In particular, blueberries have several known health benefits. They exert positive effects upon your lipid profile, reducing your risk for type II diabetes. And because of their bountiful antioxidants, blueberries are one of the best fruits to protect you from premature aging. Blueberries have also been shown to alleviate inflammatory intestinal conditions, such as ulcerative colitis.

Two recent studies reveal even more about how berries can protect you against illness. One study published in the June 2014 issue of *Cancer Immunology and Immunotherapy* identified a compound in black raspberries that suppresses the growth of tumor cells. Another recent study found that strawberries contain a compound called fisetin that may help prevent Alzheimer's disease and memory loss.

KIWIS
Kiwis are great for weight loss because they are packed full of fiber. The

black seeds combine for a good dose of insoluble fiber, which aids digestion. But kiwis also offers soluble fiber, providing bulk that promotes the feeling of fullness.

PEACHES

Peach is an ideal fruit to incorporate in low calorie diet. It contains a high amount of fiber, potassium and it is full of vitamins. Several studies have shown that peaches are a good source of antioxidants so they are great for flushing toxins from your body.

COCONUT

Coconut is a very sweet and filling snack that can satisfy your sweet tooth. You can consume it as coconut oil, water, milk, flour and even as dry fruit. It contains chains of triglycerides that raise the metabolic rate of the liver up to 30 percent, therefore helping you lose weight.

Some media reports advise you to stay clear of coconuts because they are high in saturated fats. However, scientific studies prove that the saturated fat in coconuts is completely different from the saturated fat that we all try to avoid. For example, coconut oil is a fat that is made up of medium chain fatty acids that and is not stored in our bodies as fat.

POMEGRANATE

One study from the University of Carolina proves that the polyphenols antioxidants in pomegranate boost the body's metabolism. In addition, they stop the build up of the arterial lipid and lower your appetite. It is an excellent choice of fruit when it comes to weight loss. It also reduces LDL cholesterol, removes harmful toxins and increases the blood flow in the body.

AVOCADOS

Avocados are nutritional gems, including being rich sources of monounsaturated fat that your body can easily burn for energy. Because they are so rich in healthy fats, avocados help your body absorb fat-soluble nutrients from other foods. They also provide close to 20 essential health-boosting nutrients, including potassium, vitamin E, B vitamins, and folic acid.

A recent study published in *The Journal of Nutrition* found that consuming a whole fresh avocado with either an orange-colored tomato sauce or raw carrots significantly enhanced your body's absorption of the carotenoids and conversion of them into an active form of vitamin A.

The greatest concentration of beneficial carotenoids is in the dark green flesh of the avocado, closest to the peel, so you're best off peeling your avocado with your hands, like a banana. Avocados have the following additional health benefits:

They reduce excess cholesterol;

They reduce inflammation;

They fight cancer cells;

They protect your liver; and,

They help with weight management. According to a recent study, if you are overweight, eating just one-half of a fresh avocado with lunch may satiate you and reduce excessive snacking.

LEMONS

Lemons are an excellent liver detoxifier. Drink a glass of lemon juice and water first thing in the morning to prevent fat accumulation and squeeze liberally over you cooked food and salads.

CUCUMBERS

The humble cucumber is one of the best vegetables for weight loss. They are extremely low in calories and contain 95 per cent water. They also contain a number of necessary vitamins and minerals, as well as exerting anti-inflammatory properties. They are rich in vitamin B5 (pantothenic acid), fisetin, vitamin C, vitamin K, potassium, magnesium, manganese, silica, and fiber, and can help your body eliminate toxins.

Recent studies show that they also contain powerful lignans that bind with estrogen-related bacteria in the digestive tract to potentially reduce your risk of breast, uterine, ovarian, and prostate cancer. Their anti-inflammatory properties make them useful when applied topically for skin irritations and puffiness, and are excellent for sunburn and puffy eyes. Traditionally, cucumbers have been used to treat headaches and water retention. As well as being served up in salads, cucumber can also be grilled.

BROCCOLI

Broccoli contains no fat at all, and plenty of slow-release carbohydrates, which is great for helping to keep your energy levels up. In addition to warding off prostate, breast, lung and skin cancers, it helps you lose weight. It contains a phytonutrient called sulforaphane that increase testosterone and fights off body fat storage. It's also rich in vitamin C. Does it have any downside? Yes, it can give you wind but besides that it is one of the top super foods out there.

SPINACH

Spinach is another excellent choice of vegetable if you're trying to lose weight. It can actually help take your calorie-burning potential to the next level. How? The green is overflowing with protein, a nutrient that aids post-pump muscle recovery and growth. And remember that the more muscle mass you have, the more calories you burn while resting. In addition, it is rich in thylakoids, a compound that's been shown to significantly reduce cravings and promote weight loss. Why do you think Popeye ate so much?

CARROTS

Carrots are another must have vegetable for losing weight. Full of beta-carotene and fiber and delicious raw.

CELERY

Like cucumber, celery is pretty much all water, and contains hardly any calories, so it's great for weight loss. It is also packed with fiber and protein as well. Delicious raw, just exclude the creamy dip!

SWEET AND CHILI PEPPERS

Sweet peppers are excellent for weight loss because they are sweet and can help lose those sweet cravings. They're great for providing vitamin C. Thanks to a metabolism-boosting compound, dihydrocapsiate, and their high vitamin-C content, sweet red and green peppers can help you lose weight. A cup of these bell-shaped veggies serves up to three times the day's recommended vitamin C.

Chili peppers are also useful on a weight loss diet. They contain a substance called capsaicin, which has been shown to help reduce appetite and increase fat burning in some studies. This substance is often sold in supplement form in many commercial weight loss programs. One study showed that eating 1 gram of red chili pepper reduced appetite and increased fat burning in people who didn't regularly eat peppers. However, there was no effect in people who were accustomed to eating spicy food.

ONIONS

Onions are rich in quercetin, which is a flavonoid that increase blood flow and activates a protein in the body. This assists in regulating glucose levels. It also eliminates stored fat and keeps new fat cells from forming. Simply speaking, onions are the unsung hero of cardiovascular health. They can help lower cholesterol, ward off hardening of the arteries and help maintain healthy blood-pressure levels. But the best part of all is that they are super low-cal and go with just about anything.

MUSHROOMS

Used for centuries in Eastern medicine these tasty, versatile vegetable have powerful effects on the immune system. This is especially so in the maitake, shiitake, and reishi varieties. In fact, mushrooms, particularly the maitake variety, can help prevent and treat cancer, viral diseases, high cholesterol, and high blood pressure.

They are used as an adjunctive cancer treatment throughout Asia because of their ability to counteract the toxic effects of chemotherapy and radiation while at the same time shrinking tumors. Japanese researchers have shown that regularly eating shiitake mushrooms lowers blood cholesterol levels up to 45 percent.

CABBAGE

Part of the Brassica family, cabbage like broccoli, contains compounds called indoles, which have been shown to reduce the risk of cancer dramatically. Studies show that eating cabbage more than once a week cut men's colon cancer odds by 66 percent. It also stimulates the immune system, kills bacteria and viruses, and is a good blood purifier. If you eat red cabbage you'll also get a healthy dose of anthocyanins (the same pigment molecules that make blueberries blue), another powerful antioxidant with an anticancer punch.

GARLIC

Studies show that garlic lowers total cholesterol and triglyceride (blood fat) levels, helping prevent clogged arteries. Two to three cloves a day cut the odds of subsequent heart attacks in half for heart disease patients. It also tops the National Cancer Institute's list of potential cancer-preventive foods.

Whole baked garlic helps detoxify the body of heavy metals like mercury (from fish) and cadmium. It also acts as an antibacterial and antiviral, boosting resistance to stress-induced colds and infections. OK, it's not a huge weight loss vegetable but I thought I should mention it anyway.

POTATOES

White potatoes seems to have fallen out of favor in recent years with health commentators extolling the virtues of sweet potatoes and propelling them into the super food stratosphere but let's not forget the simple white potato.

White potatoes have the properties that make them a perfect food, both for weight loss and optimal health. They contain an incredibly diverse range of nutrients, a little bit of almost everything we need. There have even been accounts of people living on nothing but potatoes alone for extended periods of time.

They are particularly high in potassium, a nutrient that most people don't get enough of and plays an important role in blood pressure control. On a scale called the Satiety Index, that measures how fulfilling different foods are, white boiled potatoes scored the highest of all the foods tested.

What this means is that by eating white, boiled potatoes, you will naturally feel full and eat less of other foods instead. If you boil the potatoes, then allow them to cool for a while, then they will form large amounts of resistant starch, a fiber-like substance that has been shown to have all sorts of health benefits... including weight loss.

If you typically eat your potatoes warm out of the oven, you're missing out on the spud's fat-fighting superpowers. When you throw potatoes in the refrigerator and eat them cold, their digestible starches turn into resistant starches through a process called retrogradation. As the name implies, resistant starch, well, resists digestion, which promotes fat oxidation and reduces abdominal fat. Sweet potatoes, turnips and other root vegetables are also excellent.

SEAWEED
Seaweed is now the ultimate superfood. Scientists at the University of Newcastle upon Tyne in England have carried out research on alginate, a substance found in brown seaweed. Their studies proved that it can strengthen gut mucus which protects the gut wall and slow down digestion so you feel fuller for longer.

It also makes food release its energy more slowly and is high in fiber. Meanwhile, a recent Japanese study shows that high seaweed intake increases the good bacteria in the gut. Wakeme is a form of seaweed. A study reported in the British *Journal of Nutrition* states that wakeme is an excellent source of calcium, iodine, folate and magnesium, while purple laver is especially rich in B vitamins.

Another report in the same journal states that wakeme prevents high blood pressure in animals while research from Kyoto University showed that the fibers from brown seaweed lowered blood pressure and reduced the risk of stroke in animals predisposed to cardiovascular problems.

Seaweed is very high in lignans. These are plant substances that become phytoestrogens in the body, which help to block the chemical oestrogens that can predispose people to cancers such as breast cancer. Dr. Jane Teas of Harvard University published a paper saying that kelp consumption might be a factor in lowering rates of breast cancer in Japan.

She is now researching the effects of seaweed as a natural replacement for HRT. Several studies indicate it is also an excellent vegetable for weight loss. Just make sure you buy it from a reputable source.

BEETROOT

Don't forget beetroot. Calorie density, or energy density, is the measurement of calories per weight of food. Eating food with a low calorie density will make you feel full on fewer calories. Half a cup of sliced cooked beets contains just 37 calories. So, are they good for losing weight? Beets contain no cholesterol or fat and are packed with nutrition.

In fact, they provide 6% daily value for vitamin C and 2 % DV for calcium. Beets contain 55 milligrams of sodium per half cup, which is 2% of our daily recommended value. According to the National Institute of Health in America, beets are rich in folate, which prevents birth defects such as spina bifida, heart and brain abnormalities.

Jennifer Di Noia is an associate professor of sociology at William Paterson University. She recently carried out a study to ascertain which fruit and vegetables contain the most nutrients. She concentrated on 17 nutrients considered by experts to be the most important for good health and for lowering risk of heart disease and cancer. The nutrients were potassium, fiber, protein, calcium, iron, thiamin, riboflavin, niacin, folate, zinc, and vitamins A, B6, B12, C, D, E, and K.

Her table is shown on the following page.

ITEM	NUTRIENT DENSITY SCORE
Watercress	99.99
Chinese cabbage	91.99
Chard	89.27
Beet green	87.08
Spinach	86.43
Chicory	73.36
Leaf lettuce	70.73
Parsley	65.59
Romaine lettuce	63.48
Collard green	62.49
Turnip green	62.12
Mustard green	61.39
Endive	60.44
Chive	54.80
Kale	49.07
Dandelion green	46.34
Red pepper	41.26
Arugula	37.65
Broccoli	34.89
Pumpkin	33.82
Brussels sprout	32.23
Scallion	27.35
Kohlrabi	25.92
Cauliflower	25.13
Cabbage	24.51
Carrot	22.60
Tomato	20.37
Lemon	18.72
Iceberg lettuce	18.28
Strawberry	17.59
Radish	16.91
Winter squash (all varieties)	13.89
Orange	12.91
Lime	12.23
Grapefruit (pink and red)	11.64
Rutabaga	11.58
Turnip	11.43
Blackberry	11.39
Leek	10.69
Sweet potato	10.51
Grapefruit (white)	10.47

RULE #3. EAT MORE EGGS

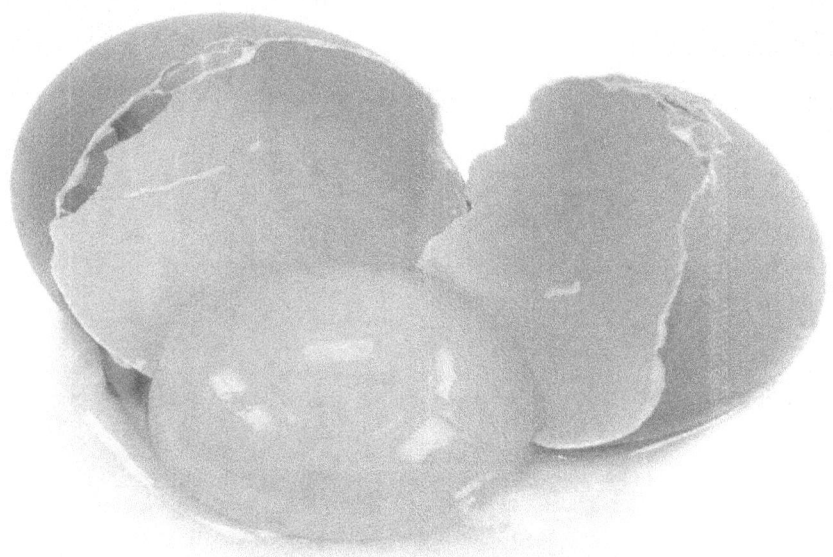

Eggs are pretty much the perfect superfood. They have so many benefits but the one that is most important to you is that they help you lose weight. A 2005 study from the Rochester Centre for Obesity in America [1] showed that by eating eggs for breakfast (rather than bagels) could help to limit your calorie intake throughout the rest of the day, by more than 400 calories.

In the study, 30 overweight or obese women ate either an egg-based breakfast containing two eggs or a bagel-based breakfast, containing the same amount of calories and almost identical levels of protein. The research studied the women's eating habits and discovered that just before lunch, the women who had eaten eggs for breakfast felt less hungry and ate a smaller lunch as a result. Even better was the fact that over the next thirty six hours the egg eating group consumed, on average, 417 calories less than the bagel-eating group.

The study suggests that eating eggs for breakfast makes you feel fuller for longer so that you eat less at your next few meals. This is excellent news if you're trying to lose weight as it means you may find it easier to cut calories without feeling hungry. In fact, based on these results you could expect to lose up to 2 lb a month, simply by eating eggs for breakfast!

In a similar study [2], three years later, published in the *International Journal of Obesity*, 152 overweight men and women were split into groups. Like the 2005 study, one group ate eggs, the other ate bagels. Both groups were on a weight loss diet for eight weeks. After that period the egg group had lost significantly more weight than the bagel group:
•65% more weight loss (2 lbs vs 1.3 lbs).
•61% greater reduction in BMI.
•34% greater reduction in waist circumference.
•16% greater reduction in body fat percentage.

While the difference in weight loss was not massive the study clearly demonstrates that simple things like changing one meal can have a small effect. Eggs are packed with a variety of nutrients including protein, zinc, iron and vitamins A, D, E and B12, but contain just 85 calories each. You've probably read somewhere that you should limit your intake of eggs to just a few per week. Forget that.

According to the American Food Standards Agency, there is now no limit to the number of eggs you can eat in a week as part of a healthy balanced diet. Most current experts now agree that you can eat three eggs a day, every day. Also, you can forget what you read about eggs raising your cholesterol or giving you heart disease. The studies outlined below prove that both of these assertions are utter myth. Eggs are the perfect food and here are the scientifically proved reasons why.

WHAT ABOUT CHOLESTEROL?
Let's deal with the cholesterol issue first. It is true that eggs are high in cholesterol? In fact, a single egg contains 212 mg, which is over half of the recommended daily intake of 300 mg. However, it's important to remember that cholesterol in the diet does not necessarily raise cholesterol in the blood. The liver actually produces large amounts of cholesterol every single day (unless, of course, it is damaged due to excessive intakes of alcohol).

When we eat more eggs, the liver just produces less cholesterol instead, so it tends to even it out.

But the effects of egg consumption vary between individual:
In 70% of people, eggs don't raise cholesterol at all.
In the other 30% who are called "hyper responders", eggs can mildly raise Total and LDL cholesterol. LDL stands for Low Density Lipoprotein often referred to as the bad cholesterol.

It gets a bit complicated but I will show you that these changes are actually beneficial. There are exceptions to this rule. People with genetic disorders like familial hypercholesterolemia or a gene type called ApoE4 may want to minimize or avoid eggs altogether. The important thing to remember is that while eggs are high in cholesterol, eating eggs does not adversely effect cholesterol in the blood for the vast majority of people.

In actual fact, eggs raise our good cholesterol. HDL stands for High Density Lipoprotein. People who have higher levels of HDL usually have a lower risk of heart disease, stroke and various health problems. Eating eggs is a great way to increase HDL. Studies show that eating just two eggs per day for six weeks increased HDL levels by 10% .

Finally, on the cholesterol issue, it has been proven that having high levels of LDL is linked to an increased risk of heart disease. But what many people don't realize is that there are subtypes of LDL that have to do with the size of the particles. There are small, dense LDL particles and then there are large LDL particles. Several studies show that those with predominantly small, dense LDL particles have a higher risk of heart disease than people who have mostly large LDL particles.

So, even if eggs tend to mildly raise LDL cholesterol in some people, there is abundant evidence to prove that the particles change from small, dense to large LDL and, trust me, this is a good thing. To summarize, egg consumption appears to change the pattern of LDL particles from small, dense LDL (bad) to large LDL, which is linked to a reduced heart disease risk.

NUTRITION
Eggs are incredibly nutritious. Remember, a whole egg contains all the nutrients required to turn a single cell into a baby chicken. In fact, a single large boiled egg contains:
Vitamin A: 6% of the RDA.
Folate: 5% of the RDA.

Vitamin B5: 7% of the RDA.
Vitamin B12: 9% of the RDA.
Vitamin B2: 15% of the RDA.
Phosphorus: 9% of the RDA.
Selenium: 22% of the RDA.
Eggs also contain decent amounts of Vitamin D, Vitamin E, Vitamin K, Vitamin B6, Calcium and Zinc

Furthermore, eggs contain various other trace nutrients that are important for health, basically, a little bit of almost every nutrient we need. Things are even better if you have access to Omega-3 enriched eggs. They have more Omega-3s and are much higher in vitamin A and E (2, 3). Which brings me to the point that not all eggs are created equally. Some are better than others.

The nutrient composition of eggs varies depending on how the hens were fed and raised. Eggs from hens that are raised on pasture and/or fed Omega-3 enriched feeds tend to be much higher in Omega-3 fatty acids. Omega-3 fatty acids are known to reduce blood levels of triglycerides, a well known risk factor for heart disease. Research has shown that consuming Omega-3 enriched eggs is a very effective way to reduce triglycerides in the blood. In one such study, just 5 omega-3 enriched eggs per week for 3 weeks reduced triglycerides by between 16-18% . So, if you can get them eat Omega 3 eggs.

WHAT ABOUT HEART DISEASE?
The truth is that eggs do not raise your risk of heart disease. In fact, they may even reduce the risk of a stroke. A proliferation of recent studies have examined the relationship between egg consumption and the risk of heart disease. One study [3] published in the *British Medical Journal* in 2013 examined seventeen different studies with a total of 263,938 participants.

They found no evidence of an association between egg consumption and heart disease or stroke. Many other studies have led to the same conclusion BUT some studies have found that people with diabetes who eat eggs have an increased risk of heart disease.

Whether it is the eggs that are actually causing the increased risk isn't known, because these types of studies can only show statistical association. The studies can not prove that eggs caused anything. It could well be that diabetics who eat eggs are less health conscious.

Other studies show that on a low-carb diet, which is by far the best diet for diabetics, eating eggs leads to improvements in risk factors for heart disease. In summary, while many studies have looked at egg consumption and the risk of heart disease and found no association, some have found an increased risk in people with type II diabetes.

CHOLINE

Have you ever heard of Choline? It's an important nutrient often grouped with the B vitamins. Choline is used to build cell membranes. It also helps to produce signaling molecules in the brain, along with various other functions. Dietary surveys in America have shown that about 90% of Americans are not getting the recommended amount of choline. Whole eggs are an excellent source of choline. A single egg contains more than 100 mg of this very important nutrient.

You may not have heard of Lutein or Zeaxanthin. These are antioxidants that hold major benefits for eye health. As we get older our eyesight deteriorates. There are several nutrients that help counteract some of the degenerative processes that can affect our eyes. Two of these are Lutein and Zeaxanthin.

These are powerful antioxidants that tend to build up in the retina of the eye. Research has proved that consuming adequate amounts of these nutrients can significantly reduce the risk of cataracts and macular degeneration which are two very common eye disorders. This brings us to eggs. Egg yolks actually contain large amounts of both Lutein and Zeaxanthin.

A 1999 controlled trial [4], published in the *American Society for Clinical Nutrition* showed that eating just 1.3 egg yolks per day for 4.5 weeks increased blood levels of Lutein by 28-50% and Zeaxanthin by 114-142%.

Furthermore, eggs are also high in vitamin A and a deficiency in this vitamin is the most common cause of blindness in the world.

Finally, eggs are high in quality protein and contain all the essential amino acids in the correct ratios. Proteins are used to make all sorts of tissues and molecules that serve both structural and functional purposes. Accordingly, getting enough protein in the diet is hugely important.

Recent studies suggest that currently recommended amounts may be too low. The solution? Eat more eggs. Eggs are an excellent source of protein, with a single large egg containing 6 grams. And as eggs contain all the essential amino acids in the right ratios, our bodies are well equipped to make full use of the protein in them. Eating adequate protein can assist us in losing weight, increase muscle mass, lower blood pressure and optimize bone health.

So, the bottom line is try and eat three Omega 3 eggs a day.

References:

[1] *The Short-term effect of eggs on satiety in overweight and obese subjects.*

[2] *Egg Breakfast Enhances Weight Loss.*

[3] *Egg Consumption and Risk of Coronary Heart Disease and Stroke: Dose-response Meta-analysis of Prospective Cohort Studies.*

[4] *Lutein and Zeaxanthin Concentrations in Plasma after Dietary Supplementation with Egg Yolks*

RULE #4. USE GLUCOMANNAN AS A FOOD SUPPLEMENT

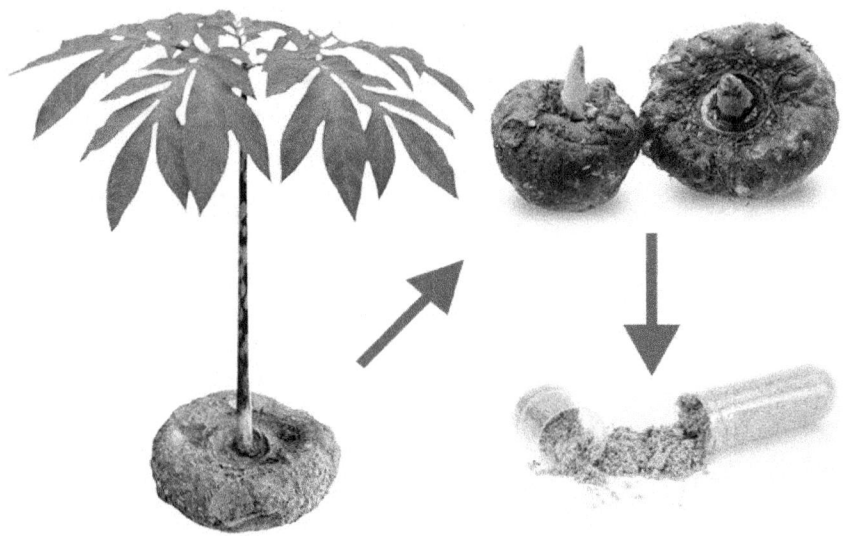

New weight-loss supplements are coming out all the time and it's difficult to know which ones work and which don't. According to nutrition expert Dr. Oz, Glucomannan, the so-called miracle supplement, is the one to use. It's basically a natural thickening agent. Oz says it is an excellent way to control your hunger because it is the best appetite suppressant on the market. Is he right?

What exactly is it? Glucomannan is a sugar made agent from the root of the konjac plant. It has been used for centuries in traditional Japanese cooking as a thickener or gelling agent. It's so well known in Japan that they call it "the broom of the intestines". This should give you a pretty good idea of how it works. For just a few calories it creates a sense of fullness by absorbing water in the system and expanding to form a bulky fiber in your stomach. Essentially, it likes like a sponge, soaking up the water in the digestive tract, reducing the absorption of carbs and cholesterol and accordingly supporting weight loss. It actually makes you feel full without leaving you feel full of gas or bloated.

The result is that this "bulky fiber" is then expelled from your body by its natural route. This cleansing effect has been said to help people reduce their cholesterol, control blood sugar in people with type II diabetes, and assist with constipation problems. But does it really work?

While America's FDA has not yet given its approval to any glucomannan product's health or weight loss claims, preliminary studies are promising. In 2008, a study [1] was published in the British *Journal of Nutrition*. The study showed that participants taking a glucomannan and psyllium husk combination supplement lost approximately 10 pounds in 16 weeks compared to 1.7 pounds lost in the placebo group.

Another 1984 study [2], published in the *International Journal of Obesity* held that participants using only glucomannan showed an average of 5.5 pounds lost over eight weeks, without making any other diet or lifestyle changes.

So, how do you take it and where do you get it? It's a supplement and you can get in a powder form or in tablet form it in any good health shop. It contains no harsh chemicals, strange drugs, or additives, so it is considered "likely safe" to use as an appetite suppressant. However, there are a few side effects that you need to look out for.

First and foremost, you need to be careful that you drink enough water. Most experts advise that you take 8 ounces of water with 1 gram of glucomannan before each meal. If you don't drink enough, the fiber will clog up your digestive system. This could result in intestinal blockages and, in rare cases, choking by blocking your throat. Also, as one woman's "cleanse" is another woman's date-night disaster my advice is to start slowly and work your way up to to the full dosage to see how your body deals with it.

I recommend that you take it (with water) 15-30 minutes before a meal. The powder form is virtually tasteless. It's a perfect supplement to add to smoothies and it gives them a nice thick consistency. But perhaps the easiest way is to take them in tablet form. Always read the label carefully.

The bottom line is that this food suppressant supplement is a great way to lose weight.

References:

[1] *The Effect of two doses of a mixture of soluble fibres on body weight and metabolic variables in overweight or obese patients: a randomised trial.*

[2] *The Effect of glucomannan on obese patients: a clinical study.*

RULE #5. ENJOY THE BENEFITS OF PROBIOTICS

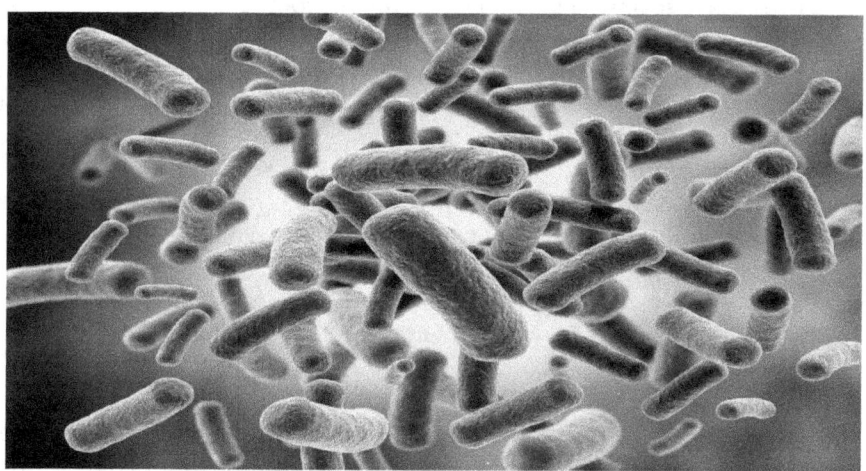

Can probiotics help you lose weight? On first glance the scientific evidence would say yes. Personally speaking, I'm not yet convinced so you can make up your own mind from what I have extracted from the scientific evidence. One thing is a given, probiotics are excellent for your general health.

WHAT ARE PROBIOTICS?

The official definition states they are "live microorganisms that, when administered in adequate amounts, confer a health benefit on the host." Basically, they are foods or supplements that contain friendly bacteria. They are designed to help colonize our guts with health-boosting microorganisms. This is hugely important because taking care of your gut and the friendly bacteria that reside there, may be one of the single most important things you can do for your health.

Don't confuse probiotics with prebiotics. Prebiotics are dietary fibers that help feed the friendly bacteria that are already in the gut. Actually, there are dozens of different probiotic bacteria that are known to have health benefits. The most common groups include Lactobacillus and Bifidobacterium. Then there are many different species within each group. Each species has many strains.

Evidence suggests that different probiotics work for different health conditions. Therefore, choosing the right type (or types) of probiotic is absolutely crucial. You can obtain probiotics from supplements, as well as foods that are prepared by bacterial fermentation. Probiotic foods include yogurt, kefir, sauerkraut, kimchi and tempeh. Several probiotic supplements combine different species together in the same supplement. These are known as broad-spectrum probiotics, or multi-probiotics.

Current research finds new benefits tied to these tiny bacteria almost on a monthly basis but the question you want answered is whether or not probiotics can help you lose weight. Recent research has shown probiotics can aid digestion and ward off illness. And a recent study, published in the British *Journal of Nutrition*, links one probiotic strain to fat loss. But can you trust these weight-reduction claims? In one study, a team of Japanese researchers split 210 overweight people into three groups. While each participant consumed a daily 7-ounce serving of fermented milk, two of the groups drank milk spiked with varying amounts of the probiotic called Lactobacillus gasseri SBT2055.

This particular probiotic has, in the past, been linked to weight loss. After 12 weeks, people consuming the probiotic milk formulas dropped roughly 8 to 9% of their visceral fat. Visceral fat is a particularly unhealthy type of fat that builds up around your heart and organs. The study also showed that both probiotic groups also lost 1 to 3% of their belly fat.

As you probably know your intestines manage the digestion and absorption of the foods you eat and it's possible the probiotic featured in this study does lower intestinal inflammation, aids digestion and prevents the build up of body fat. However, there are problems.

Firstly, the particularly probiotic strain highlighted in this research isn't commercially available.

Secondly, the majority of the research linking probiotics to weight loss have been conducted or funded by companies who sell products containing those same probiotics. Now, don't get me wrong. I'm not saying that the research isn't valid, but I am wondering just how independent it is. As Dr. Jeremy Burton, deputy director of the Canadian Research and Development Centre for Probiotics says: "There's nothing wrong with companies investing in studies, but it's better when the study is backed up by independent research."

To date, that independent research is either inconclusive or contradictory. A study published in the *International Journal of Obesity* found that while some strains of probiotics aid weight loss, others contribute to obesity. When I questioned Dr. Didier Raoult, a Marseille, France-based microbiologist who is co-author of the study about the results he admitted that the research now is premature, and requires more analysis. So, the jury's still out on probiotics when it comes to weight loss.

Maybe, I'm been too picky. In the last few years, researchers have discovered particular bacterial strains that can ease irritable bowel syndrome (IBS) and help prevent and treat vaginal yeast infections. And preliminary research indicates that other strains may help improve vascular health, battle depression, and even ward off cancer.

Research discoveries are only in their embryonic stages and it is possible that, in the not too distant future, probiotics may be used in prescription drugs to treat a range of conditions, from acne to depression. While probiotics are by no means a magic super drug, many experts feel they're especially useful when your body's normal bacterial balance is interrupted. This can occur when we are stressed, ill, traveling, or taking antibiotics.

There is no doubt that yogurt manufacturers have an interest in plugging probiotics. According to the Specialty Food Association, an astonishing $2.27 billion worth of yogurt and kefir, a fermented milk drink, were sold in the U.S. in 2012. So what is the best probiotic for you? In my opinion, the best, most natural forms of probiotics are fermented foods. Fortified foods, like probiotic-enhanced dough, may deliver less of a health infusion since the manufacturing process can kill off many of the healthy live cultures. Besides yogurt and kefir, some common foods made using fermentation include sauerkraut, kimchi (spicy pickled cabbage), and pickles.

The amount and kind of live cultures per bite vary. You need to look out for words like raw, lacto-fermented, or unpasteurized on the packaging as this will indicate that the bacteria haven't been killed off in the manufacturing process. Any yogurt with a "live active cultures" seal indicates that it has not been heated after the fermentation process and contains at least 100 million cultures per gram (or 10 million cultures per gram for frozen yogurt). However, I should point out that unless it contains one of the bacterial strains that have been studied, it still may not have proven probiotic benefits.

The following brands may be worth trying.

DanActive: Some research suggests that it can help ease some types of gastrointestinal distress.

Lifeway Frozen Kefir: Kefir can improve digestion and restore beneficial bacteria particularly after a round of antibiotics.

Mama O's Premium Kimchi: Lactobacilli, found in kimchi, can help prevent yeast infections. Real Pickles Organic Sauerkraut: A study published in the British *Journal of Nutrition* found that eating sauerkraut may help prevent cancer.

Align: It contains Bifantis, which helps maintain digestive balance.

Florastor: A study found it alleviates antibiotic-related diarrhea and may help aid the immune system, so it's a good supplement to take when travelling.

RepHresh Pro-B: This is the only probiotic clinically shown to balance yeast and bacteria daily.

Dr. Frank Lipman's Be Well Probiotic Powder: This can help for chronic indigestion and bloating. Add a teaspoon to your smoothie or mix with water.

Culturelle Digestive Health Probiotic Chewables: These have been shown to boost general digestive health.

RULE #6. EAT MORE FISH

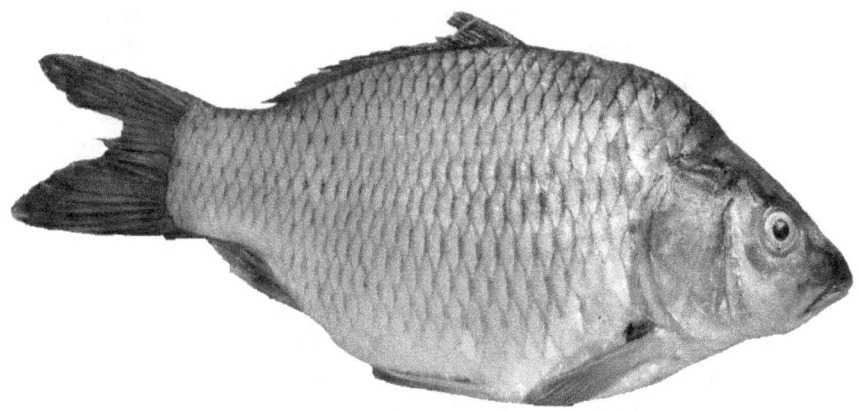

We already know that if you are embarking on a weight loss diet that a good source of lean protein relatively low in calories is essential. Many people consume chicken and lean meat in such diets but switching over to fish is a better choice. Fish is hugely nutritious. Although certain varieties may be considered 'fatty' or 'oily', unlike red meat, they are high in healthy omega 3 fatty acids and low in unhealthy saturated fats. Fish oil and omega 3 fatty acids are linked to several health benefits, including lowering blood triglycerides, reducing risk of heart disease as well as possible benefits for a huge range of illnesses from arthritis to stroke.

According to a 2002 report [1] endorsed by the American Heart Association Science Advisory and Coordinating Committee, mega-3 fatty acids appear to be especially important for mental health and prevention of cardiovascular disease.

Another study published in the *Journal of Clinical Psychiatry* in 2007 claims that Omega-3's are very beneficial for depression, which means that eating fish one to two times per week may literally make you feel better every single day. Another plus in eating fish is that its consumption helps to keep your skin looking young. Eating fish high in omega-3s can help keep your skin-cell membranes strong and elastic. Omega 3s are also beneficial for people with sensitivity to the sun.

The bottom line is that we should all include fish in our diets and try and eat it at least twice per week. So, we know it is good for us. But can it help us lose weight? In a word, yes.

Studies show, that as part of a calorie controlled weight loss diet, fish and fish oil will enhance weight loss. How come? Well, this may be because fish is generally lower in calories than the red meat that it might replace in an average diet. So, a larger quantity can be eaten for the same amount of calories. This may help to keep you fuller for longer.

As Omega 3 fatty acids from oily fish or fish oil supplementation have also been associated with better weight loss in a number of studies, it can be positively concluded that fish plays a valuable part in a healthy weight loss diet.

Does the type of fish you eat make a difference? In 2007 the *International Journal of Obesity* published a study which suggested that the type of fish was not particularly important when it came to enhanced weight loss. The study in overweight males compared weight loss after following a calorie restricted diet over the course of four weeks.

Four groups received the same amount of calories, but one group had a diet free of seafood, another with oily fish, the third with lean fish and the final group with fish oil supplements. It was found that over the four weeks that the groups who ate both types of fish and the fish oil lost approximately 1 kg more than the seafood free group. This suggests that any type of fish may have some effect on weight loss when combined with an energy restricted diet.

Other studies have associated omega 3 fatty acids, which are more prevalent in oily fish, with weight loss. Fish oil may also help with weight loss. However, it is better to eat the whole fish (fileted) due to the extra nutrients that are present and the protein that can help with satiety levels.

Certain fish are overall more healthy to eat than others. Also, it is important to remember that to achieve effective weight loss you should not eat fish cooked in batter, in copious amount of butter or fish that is deep fried. It's better to grill it lightly and serve it with lemon butter or simply steam it. As with all food, some fish are better than others. The following fish are considered to be the most healthy: cod, halibut, salmon, sardines, herring, anchovies, rainbow trout, oysters, scallops, and tuna.

COD

Research suggests that a regular serving of Pacific cod will help you lose weight. A recent 2009 study [2] in the journal *Nutrition, Metabolism and Cardiovascular Diseases*, found that eating fish instead of other lean protein products can result in faster weight loss.

In the study, researchers split the pool of subjects into three groups: One was given lean meat as a main protein source. Another was given cod three times weekly in place of the lean meat; while a third was given cod five times per week in place of meat. The participants followed this protocol as part of a strict diet for eight weeks. Even in this short time span, researchers noticed significant differences.

According to the results, just three weekly servings of cod was enough to promote weight-loss benefits, and the advantages increased with higher fish consumption. The group which had cod five times per week enjoyed the best results. They lost about 3.74 more pounds than the lean meat only group. Waist circumference and fat mass reductions were also superior in this group.

Another study published in the *European Journal of Clinical Nutrition* found that people ate 11 percent less at dinner after having cod for lunch versus those who ate a beef lunch. Researchers attribute the satiating and slimming properties to cod's high protein content and amino acid profile, which can help regulate the metabolism.

HALIBUT

Believe or not, halibut contain almost an entire day's worth of omega 3 fatty acids and are low in fat overall. This makes them a great choice for weight loss as the low fat content also means fewer calories. They are also high in potassium and vitamin D. However, they can be high in mercury. So consumption may need to be limited in high risk groups.

An Australian study [3] published in the *European Journal of Clinical Nutrition*, ranks halibut as the number two most filling food. It is only bested only by boiled potatoes for its fullness factor.

A separate Australian study that compared the satiety of different animal proteins found a nutritionally similar white fish (flake) to be significantly more satiating than beef and chicken. Satiety following the white-fish meal also declined at a much slower rate. The researchers attributed the filling factor of white fish like halibut to its impressive protein content and influence on serotonin. Serotonin is one of the key hormones responsible for appetite signals.

SALMON

Some people are scared to eat salmon because of its relatively high calorie and fat content. However, some studies suggest that this oily fish may be one of the best for weight loss.

In one particular study, participants were divided into groups and assigned one of three equi-caloric weight loss diets. The diet of the first group, the control group, included no seafood. The diet of the second group contained lean white fish and the third salmon. All the participants lost weight. However, the third group, the salmon eaters, had the lowest fasting insulin levels and a marked reduction in inflammation.

Another study published in the *International Journal of Obesity* found that eating three 5-ounce servings of salmon per week for four weeks as part of a low-calorie diet resulted in approximately 2.2 pounds more weight lost than following a equip-calorie diet that didn't include fish. Try to eat wild salmon rather than farmed salmon. Wild salmon is leaner while farmed is plumped up on fishmeal. Furthermore, wild salmon is known to be significantly lower in cancer-linked PCBs.

Sardines, herrings and anchovies are also high in omega 3s, whether they are fresh or canned. Canned varieties are an excellent way to incorporate more fish into your diet in a convenient and cheap way. Rainbow trout contain more than a day's recommended serve of omega 3 fatty acids. They are also a good source of vitamin B12 which is important for the health of the nervous system.

OYSTERS

While scientists have as yet been unable to prove that oysters are an aphrodisiac, research have shown oysters' lesser-known potential as a natural weight loss aid. A half dozen oysters contain a mere 43 calories and provide 21% of your recommended daily allowance for iron. Iron deficiencies have been linked to a significant increase in fat gene expression. In addition to this, oysters are one of the best food sources of zinc, a mineral that works in tandem with the hormone leptin which makes you feel hungry, to regulate appetite.

Research suggests that obese people tend to have higher levels of leptin and lower levels of zinc, in comparison to their leaner colleagues.

One particular study published in the journal *Life Sciences* found supplementing with zinc could increase leptin production in obese men by 142%. Six oysters satisfy your recommended daily need of zinc by 200%.

SCALLOPS

Scallops are a high-protein, low-calorie mollusk which are good for your cholesterol. A study published in the *Journal of Food Science* found bioactive capsules made from scallop by-products to show significant anti-obesity effects. Animals fed on the capsules which contained a mixture of scallop and seaweed, over the course of 4 weeks, showed greater reductions in body weight and body fat, compared to a control group. The authors attributed this to scallop's high protein content. A scallop is 80 % protein.

A separate study which examined the effects of different proteins on adipose tissue and glucose tolerance found scallops to be the tops. Mice fed scallop protein showed lower blood cholesterol and diet-induced obesity levels compared to mice fed equi-caloric portions of casein or chicken protein.

TUNA

As a prime source of docosahexaenoic acid (DHA), tuna, particularly the canned light tuna is recognized as one of the best and most affordable fish for weight loss, especially from your belly!

One study published in the *Journal of Lipid Research* showed that omega 3 fatty acid supplementation had the profound ability to turn off abdominal fat genes. And while you'll find two types of fatty acids in cold water fish and fish oils, i.e. DHA and eicosapentaenoic acid (EPA), researchers claim DHA can be 40 to 70 % more effective than EPA at down regulating fat genes in the abdomen, preventing belly fat cells from expanding in size.

Worried about the mercury? Mercury levels in tuna vary by species. In general, the larger and leaner the fish, the higher the mercury level. According to a study in *Biology Letters*, bluefin and albacore rank among the most toxic. However, canned chunk light tuna, harvested from the smallest fish, is considered a "low mercury fish." According to the FDA's most recent guidelines it is recommended that you eat it two to three times a week.

HOW TO CHOOSE AND KEEP YOUR FISH

Unless buying canned fish always ensure your fish is as fresh as possible. Smell it. If there is a fishy smell then don't buy it. Touch it. It should be firm to the touch. Check the eyes. They should be clear, not sunken, bulgy or cloudy. The scales should be shiny and clean. The fillets should be moist. If they look dried out or are curled up at the edges then the fish is not fresh.

Fish should be cooked the day you buy it. It goes off very quickly. Whole fish lasts longer than steaks or fillets. But fish will keep fresh in the refrigerator overnight providing you store it in an airtight container over a bowl of ice. If you need to keep it longer than a day, freeze it. The quality of thawed, frozen fish is better when it freezes quickly, so freeze whole fish only if it weighs two pounds or less. Larger fish should be cut into pieces, steaks, or fillets to ensure a quick freeze. Lean fish will keep in the freezer up to six months. Fatty fish will keep for three months.

If you're buying shellfish like lobster, clams, crayfish, or oysters, it's best if they are still be alive. Live lobsters and crabs are easy to spot. Clams and oysters are trickier, though; you must be sure the shell is closed tightly or closes when you tap the shell. Enjoy!

References:

[1] *Fish Consumption, Fish Oil, Omega-3 Fatty Acids, and Cardiovascular Disease.*

[2] *Consumption of cod and weight loss in young overweight and obese adults on an energy reduced diet for 8-weeks.*

[3] *The Satiety Index of Common Foods.*

RULE # 7. COPING WITH NIGHT-TIME MUNCHIES

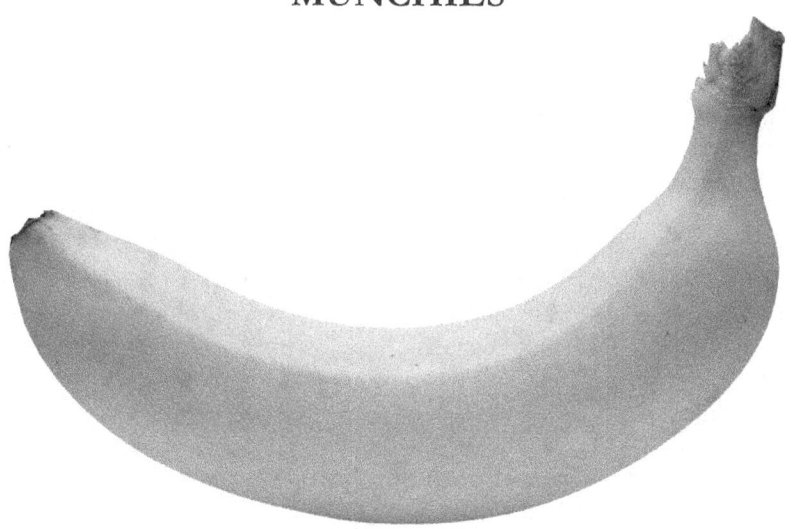

If, like me, you are one of those people who get the munchies just before bedtime then it's important to know what are the best things to eat late at night. First of all, let's dispel some myths:
A:- you can still lose weight by snacking at night.
B:- night time munchies can actually be good for you.

Studies show that small, nutrient-dense night time snacks can actually benefit metabolic health and help build muscle, especially if you exercised during the day. There are also several foods that have been proven to help us sleep better when we eat them before bed. Why is this important?

Because poor sleep is one of the strongest risk factors for obesity. The most important factor is to eat the right type of food. Here are the top five foods you can eat before sleeping which will not cause you any harm or increase your weight.

BANANA

We've already spoken about the benefits of this fruit but I never mentioned that a banana is probably the best thing to eat at night. Why? They are full of important nutrients like potassium, vitamins B6 and C and fiber. Eat a green banana because it is high in resistant starch. Studies show that fiber and resistant starch may help you feel full and less hungry. This will result in a reduction in your calorie intake. Bananas also contain the amino acid Tryptophan that helps make you sleepy. But the best thing is that a banana only has 100 calories.

TURKEY

Turkey is a relatively low-calorie meat that contains high-quality protein. Because it reduces appetite much more effectively than either fat or carbs, increasing the amount of quality protein in your diet is incredibly important for weight loss.

One 2008 study [1] published in *Regulatory Peptides* and showed that protein actually aids weight loss in two ways. Firstly, it increases calories out by raising your metabolic rate and secondly, it decreases calories in by keeping your appetite in check. Like bananas, turkey also contains high amounts of relaxing tryptophan. This is what gives it the late-night edge over other types of meat.

One 1991 study published in *Pharmacopsychiatry* found that tryptophan caused significant sleepiness, both at night and during the day. Turkey is the perfect weight-loss food because it also promotes improved sleep. High in nutrients and low in calories one or two slices at night will contain a mere 100 calories.

COTTAGE CHEESE

Yes, seriously cottage cheese is a top class food to eat at night because it actually helps build muscle while you sleep. It is another food which is high in nutrients, and tends to be low in fat and calories.

Cottage cheese is predominantly made up of a milk protein called casein. Casein is a slow-digesting protein with a reputation for sustaining overnight muscle repair and growth. What this means is that it can actively help build muscle while you sleep. A one half cup of this food provides 13 grams of protein, which is more than two boiled eggs. Cottage cheese also helps you feel full and satisfied, ensuring you go to bed with a happy stomach.

TINNED TUNA
Not only is tinned tuna an easy and filling night time snack it's also an excellent source of vitamin D. This is important considering that a massive 40% of people in America are vitamin D deficient. Vitamin D deficiency is linked to sleep disorders like worse sleep apnea. It may also decrease sleep duration. So try eating one small tin, in brine or oil, (3 ounces) at night time if you're feeling peckish. Tuna is also rich in omega-3 fats which are important for optimal body and brain function.

CHERRIES
In addition to containing only 50 calories a cup, studies show that cherries can help improve sleep, and even help treat sleep disorders. One study of people with chronic insomnia found that cherry juice greatly reduced the severity of sleeplessness. The effects were equal to or even exceeded treatment with valerian. Cherries cause a great increase in the body's secretion of the sleep hormone melatonin. In fact, cherries may actually have the greatest sleep-inducing effect of all the foods on this list.

References:

[1] *Protein intake and energy balance.*

3 WHAT TO DRINK

RULE #8. DRINK MORE WATER

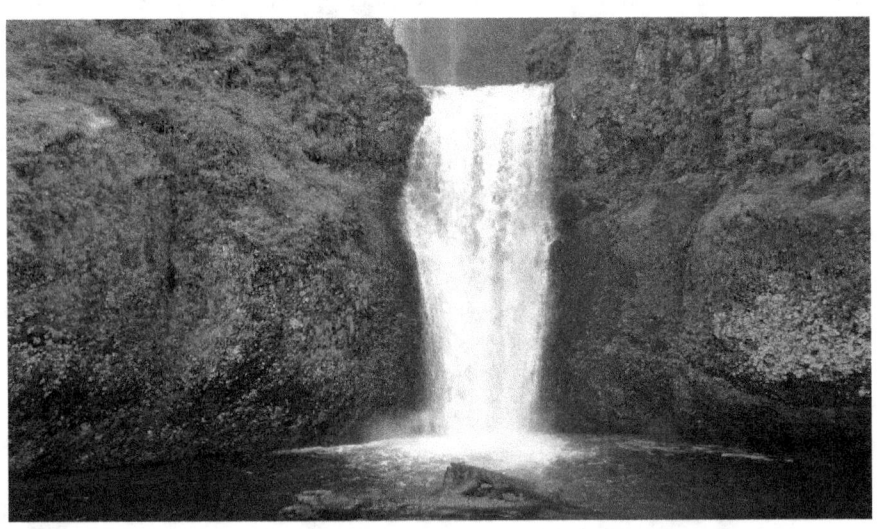

We have all heard that drinking water can help you lose weight. That's true but it's not as simple as that. Let's look at the most recent scientific evidence. In 2008, a study [1] published in the journal *Obesity*, concluded that drinking water is associated with weight loss in overweight dieting women independent of diet and activity.

A 2010 study concluded that people that consumed two cups (500 ml) of water right before eating a meal ate between 75 and 90 fewer calories during that meal. Then we had two studies in 2011. The first [2] published in the

International Journal of Obesity was conducted on obese children and concluded that water drinking on resting energy expenditure was significant.

This followed a 2007 study in which pediatricians agreed that hydration in children may be optimal only in breastfed infants. There were two significant studies in 2013. One study published in the *Journal of Clinical and Diagnostic Research* was conducted on adults aged between 18-23 and concluded that when they were given 500 ml 3 times daily for 8 weeks they lost body weight.

In August 2013 the *American Journal of Clinical Nutrition* reviewed the studies [3]. It's official. Substituting water for other drinks and drinking water before meals can help you lose weight.

Furthermore, the most recent study published in the journal *Obesity* is interesting. It showed that drinking 16 ounces of water before meals leads to more weight loss. So, if you drink a few glasses of water before you begin to eat you may eat less without even trying. The author of this study was Dr. Amanda Daley of the University of Birmingham, England. She was aware that any sort of weight management program advocated drinking lots of water to help you lose weight. Not wholly convinced by the existing studies, she and her team wanted definitive proof.

They recruited 84 adults with obesity for a 12-week experiment. Everyone was given general weight loss advice. Then they were assigned to one of two groups. The first group was told to drink 500 ml (about 16 oz) of water half an hour before their meals. The second group was told to simply imagine their stomachs were full before meals.

The researchers monitored everyone's weight at the start, middle and end of the experiment. They also checked their urine to make sure the water-boosted group was indeed drinking more water. In addition, they monitored their physical activity which didn't vary.

The first group that drank the water lost about three more pounds than the group that didn't up their water intake. And the more they drank, the better the results. Those who drank 16 ounces before every meal lost about 4.3 kg, or 9 pounds, over the course of the experiment. Daley regards that as a real success. How does it work?

Daley believes that water might be so effective because, obviously, it fills you up and helps increase satiety. She says that drinking a couple glasses of water 30 minutes before a meal gives you time to feel fuller, which can help shape decisions about what you eat. This is just a first step at getting good evidence and more research is needed before the mechanisms are fully discovered. But researchers like Dr. Amanda Daley think that drinking more water before meals can help everybody with weight management, regardless of BMI status. "We all get fatter over time, so it might well work as a prevention strategy at a population level," she says. "We want people to drink more water anyway."

So what can you do to make sure you're drinking the recommended eight-to-10 8-ounce glasses per day to keep yourself hydrated and encourage weight loss?

Drink before you eat: Because water is an appetite suppressant, drinking it before meals can make you feel fuller and therefore reduce your food intake. Health resource website WebMD states that drinking water before meals results in an average reduction in intake of 75 calories per meal. Drinking water before just one meal per day would cause you to ingest 27,000 fewer calories per year. That means that theoretically, you could lose about eight pounds per year just from drinking water.

Replace calorie-filled drinks with water: This is a no-brainer. You need to ditch the sodas and juice and replace them with water to help you lose weight. If you think water tastes boring, add a slice of lemon, mint or better still cucumber. A glass of water with lemon is a recipe for successful weight loss because the pectin in lemons helps reduce food cravings. And if you really think water doesn't really help weight loss try substituting water for those sugar filled drinks for just one week. Trust me.

Drink it ice cold: According to the editorial staff at WebMD, drinking ice cold water helps boost your metabolism because your body has to work harder to warm the water up. Therefore it helps you burn more calories and lose weight. Some claim that ice cold water is just so much more refreshing than water that's room temperature. Personally, I prefer water at room temperature because it's easier to swallow.

Ensure you drink enough: If you really want the water you drink to help you lose weight, you should follow the "8 by 8" rule recommended by most nutritionists: Drink eight 8-ounce glasses of water per day for weight loss and to maintain an ideal weight. You might need to drink more water if you exercise a lot or sweat heavily, or less water if you drink other beverages like herbal tea (make sure they are decaffeinated).

Experts like Trent Nessler from the Baptist Sports Medicine in Nashville, says the amount of water you need depends on your size, weight and activity level. He adds that you should try to drink between half an ounce and an ounce of water for each pound you weigh, every day. So, how do you know if you're getting enough water? A general rule is to check the color of your urine. If your urine is clear or very light yellow in color then you know you're well hydrated. The darker your urine, the more water you need to drink. This is especially so if you're planning to lose weight.

References:

[1] *Drinking water is associated with weight loss in overweight dieting women independent of diet and activity.*

[2] *Influence of water drinking on resting energy expenditure in overweight children.*

[3] *Association between water consumption and body weight outcomes: a systematic review.*

RULE #9. START DRINKING GREEN TEA

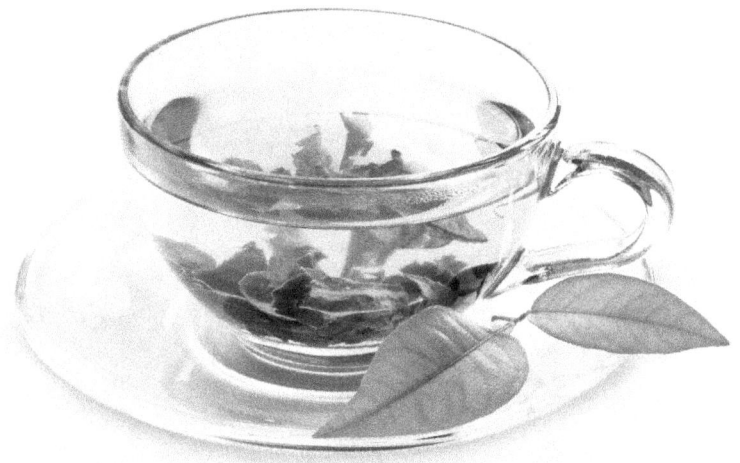

Tea is an excellent healthy drink that can help you lose weight. But, we're not talking about any kind of tea. Many Europeans, particularly the British and Irish, drink tea with milk and sugar. That beverage, as a weight loss aid, is absolutely useless. As you will see later on in the book, sugar is the worst thing you can take as part of a healthy diet. We don't need to reduce our sugar intake, we need to practically eliminate it.

Accordingly, if you think that by drinking a cup of milky tea with one or two spoons of sugar will help you lose weight then you are wrong. Black tea may be of benefit but several studies have shown that the best tea to drink is Green Tea and the best Green tea to drink is matcha. Let's investigate further.

Green tea is a natural beverage that is loaded with antioxidants. Two studies published in the *American Journal of Physiology* in 2007 and the British *Journal of Nutrition* two years earlier have shown that drinking green tea is linked with many benefits, such as increased fat burning and weight loss.

Four other studies, from 1999 to 2101 show that green tea may increase energy expenditure by 4% and increase selective fat burning by up to 17%, especially harmful belly fat.

While green tea is one of the most popular herbal tea drinks in the world matcha green tea is a variety of powdered green tea that may have even more powerful health benefits than regular green tea.

Matcha green tea is grown and prepared differently than other green teas, and the whole tea leaf is consumed. But just how good for you is it? What is matcha? Both matcha and regular green tea both come from the Camellia sinensis plant. This plant comes from China. However, matcha is grown differently than regular green tea. The tea bushes are covered for about 20–30 days before harvest. The reason for this is to protect them from direct sunlight. The shade stimulates an increase in chlorophyll levels. This turns the leaves into a darker shade of green and increases the production of amino acids.

After harvesting, the stems and veins are removed from the leaves. They are then stone-ground into a fine, bright green powder, known as matcha. Because the whole leaf powder is ingested, instead of just water infused through the tea leaves, matcha is even higher in some substances than green tea. This includes caffeine and antioxidants.

One cup of matcha, made from half a teaspoon of powder, generally contains about 35 mg of caffeine. This is slightly more than a cup of regular green tea. Matcha can have a grassy and a slightly bitter taste. In China, it is not unusual to have it served with a sweetener or milk but try to avoid these. Matcha powder is also popular in smoothies and baking.

The bottom line is that drinking two or three cups of matcha green tea everyday will help you lose weight and is seriously beneficial to your general health because it has higher amounts of caffeine and antioxidants than regular tea.

RULE #10. CUT DOWN ON COFFEE : CAFFEINE

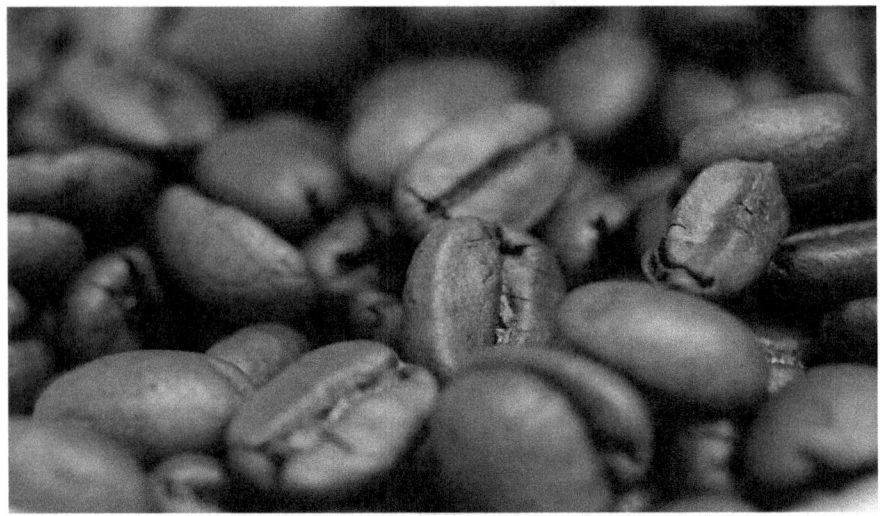

Coffee is good for you. Scratch that. Coffee is bad for you. Scratch that. Confused? Each month we seem to be confronted with another contradictory study in relation to coffee and caffeine to such an extent that it's hard to know who is right and who is wrong. Let's look at the case against coffee.

Proponents of the anti-coffee movement claim that the idea that coffee can help you lose weight is one of the great weight loss myths. They say we should not believe that the caffeine in coffee acts as an appetite suppressant and a metabolism booster. They argue that while coffee may temporarily suppress your appetite, drinking a couple of cups of coffee each day will have zero effect on helping you lose weight. They continue that four to seven cups a day will actually lead to anxiety, sleeplessness, and an increase in heart rate and blood pressure.

As an example, they cite the fact that a 16-ounce Starbucks Café Mocha can contain a whopping 330 calories. But then you've read how coffee and other forms of caffeine can help you ward off diabetes, treat headaches, control asthma, decrease the risk of getting Parkinson's disease and even help you lose weight. So who is telling the truth?

The fact is that there are over 19,000 studies examining the various benefits and downsides of ingesting caffeine. According to the Institute for Coffee Studies at Vanderbilt University, coffee is mostly beneficial. Generally, only certain groups of people (like pregnant women or people with heart disease) are warned to avoid caffeine. In other words, you don't need to give up your morning coffee. This is especially true if you're trying to lose weight fast. But, you need to be careful what you put in it. Now read on...

You've probably noticed that caffeine is a staple ingredient in many popular diet pills as well as homemade fat-burning snacks. And you've probably also heard experts suggest that you drink coffee or other caffeinated beverages to help you lose weight. All of this begs the question, can caffeine really help you lose weight?

The answer is yes, in certain circumstances. It can help you lose weight in two ways. Firstly it can help boost your metabolism. When we ingest caffeine into our system it triggers the process of lipolysis. This is the process in which your body releases free fatty acids into your bloodstream. This happens when your body is breaking down your fat stores to convert it into energy. In other words, caffeine boosts your metabolism slightly and helps you burn fat.

In fact, coffee contains at least four biologically active substances that can affect metabolism. It contains caffeine which is a central nervous system stimulant. It also contains theobromine and theophylline which are substances related to caffeine that can also have a stimulant effect. Finally, it contains chlorogenic acid. This is one of the biologically active compounds in coffee, which studies have shown may help slow absorption of carbohydrates. The most important of these is caffeine.

It also helps you lose weight by giving you an energy boost. We all know that caffeine is a stimulant. For a short period of time it will increase alertness and ward off drowsiness. This means that you can perform certain tasks for longer. These tasks are not just limited to mental tasks. They include physical tasks such as running or weight lifting. What this means is that a little shot of caffeine can give you the energy you need to give 100% during your workout. And giving 100% in the gym means you'll get the results you want more quickly.

HOW MUCH CAFFEINE?

So now that we've established that caffeine can help you with your weight loss program the next question is how much caffeine do we need? This is a more difficult question to answer since different people react to caffeine in different ways. It also depends on how much your drink. If you don't regularly ingest a lot of caffeine, then a couple hundred milligrams will likely produce noticeable effects.

You may want to start with 100 milligrams to see how it goes, then up your intake to 200 milligrams. You can then increase the dose by 50 milligrams if you're still not feeling any effects. If you don't like the taste of coffee you can ingest your caffeine in different forms, like pills, energy drinks, various foods and even shampoo and soaps.

The problem is that as coffee has considerably more caffeine than tea or chocolate and as different coffee brands and even different roasts have varying levels of caffeine it's difficult to determine exactly how much caffeine is in each cup. However, one rule of thumb is that each cup of coffee has about 80 to 125 milligrams of caffeine. It's not a bad idea to add coffee to your protein shake. But you need to be careful. Why?

Because while caffeine can boost your weight-loss efforts, it can also prejudice them. Here are some things you should not do. Firstly, do not get your daily intake of caffeine by drinking sugary or high-calorie drinks. Lattes and cappuccinos will do you more harm than good. Stick to black unsweetened coffee or even caffeine pills. Secondly, don't overdose on caffeine. Too much caffeine is bad for you. It can make your heart race, give you headaches and make you feel ill. Two or three cups a day are enough.

Don't take coffee or caffeine if you're in a "high-risk" group. People in this group include pregnant women, those with heart problems or high blood pressure. Also, studies show that the benefits of coffee decrease with age and are less prominent for obese people. My advice is that if you're not currently drinking coffee or getting caffeine in other ways, don't start. Take matcha tea instead. The bottom line is that, unless you are in the high risk group, over 60 or obese, two to three cups of black coffee a day will help you lose weight.

4 WHAT NOT TO EAT

RULE# 11. CUT OUT SUGAR

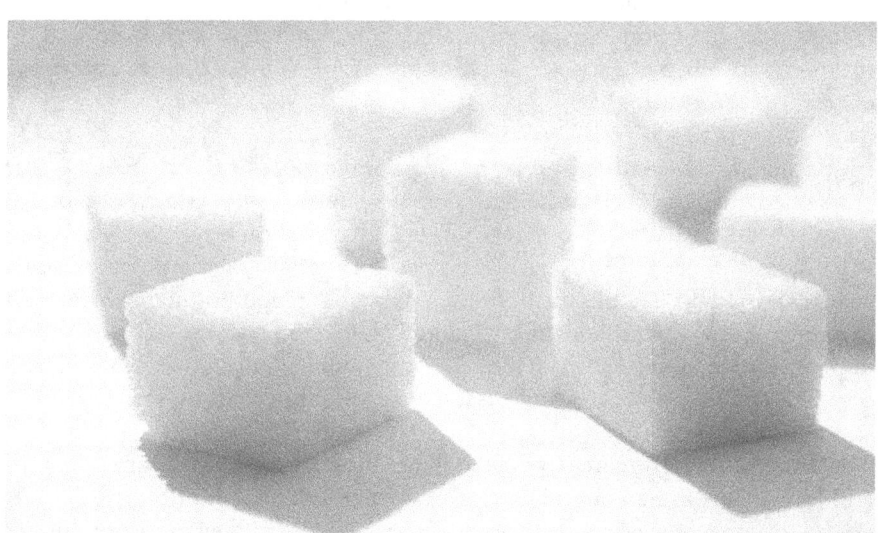

Sugar is the cancer of foods. If you were just to take one thing from this book, just one piece of advice, and act on it, then, please cut down dramatically on your sugar intake. If you take it in your tea, stop. If you take it in your coffee, stop. Why? Read on.

According to a 2015 Report by Public Health England entitled *Sugar Reduction: The evidence for action*, almost 25% of adults, 10% of 4 to 5 year olds and 19% of 10 to 11 year olds in England are obese, with significant numbers also being overweight. In 2014 around a quarter of adults were obese, that is 24% of men and 27% of women. Being overweight was more common than being obese and 41% of men and 31% of women were overweight, but not obese. Obese is defined as a Body Mass Index (BMI kg/m2) of 30 or more while overweight is defined as a Body Mass Index (BMI kg/ m2) from 25 to less than 30. Treating obesity and its consequences alone currently costs the British National Health Service over £5 billion every year.

Sugar intakes of all population groups are above the recommendations, contributing between 12 to 15% of energy. Consumption of sugar and sugar sweetened drinks is particularly high in school age children. It also tends to be highest among the most disadvantaged who also experience a higher prevalence of tooth decay and obesity and its health consequences.

Over the last 30 to 40 years there have been profound changes in our relationship with food. This includes how we shop and where we eat as well as the foods available and how they are produced. Food is now more readily available, more heavily marketed, promoted and advertised and, in real terms, is much cheaper than ever before. All of these factors encourage us towards over-eating.

In Britain, the Scientific Advisory Committee on Nutrition (SACN) has concluded that the recommended average population maximum intake of sugar should be halved. They recommend that it should not exceed 5% of total dietary energy. SACN also recommended that consumption of sugar sweetened drinks should be minimized by both adults and children. By meeting these recommendations within 10 years we would not only improve an individual's quality of life but could save the National Health Service, based on a conservative assessment, around £500m every year.

The British Government have already accepted SACN's recommendations and these recommendations are now being integrated into official UK advice on the best dietary approach for health and key nutrition policy instruments.

According to a 2015 report [1] by the Scientific Advisory Committee on Nutrition consuming too much sugar and too many foods and drinks high in sugar can lead to weight gain. This in turn can lead to an increase in the risk of heart disease, type II diabetes, stroke and even some cancers. According to a 1989 Government report it is also linked to tooth decay.

The Sugar Reduction 2015 Report clearly states: "We are eating too much sugar and it is bad for our health." The Report is convinced of sugar's link to obesity. As part of the report it published guidelines on sugar consumption.

The maximum daily recommended intake of sugar for people over the age of 11 is no more than 30g which is 7 cubes or 6-7 teaspoons. Just to put it in perspective: if you think a vanilla latte and a blueberry muffin are harmless enough, think again. Together they provide more than the total daily intake of added sugars recommended for adults.

In January 2016, Cancer Research UK and the UK Health Forum urged action to reduce the sugar intake of children and teenagers after its study found that not only could 700,000 new cases of cancer be linked to obesity and excess weight over the next 20 years, but so could millions of cases of type II diabetes, coronary heart disease and stroke. A third of children aged 10 to 11 are already above a healthy weight.

Public health statistics consistently show that this trend often continues into adulthood. The problem with sugar has become so worrying that the British government recently embarked on several campaigns to persuade and even force people to reduce their sugar intake.

These campaigns all acknowledge that there is no magic solution to this growing problem and that it requires a combination of measures. But the one step they seem to agree on is a tax on sugary drinks. In fact, Ireland may be the first European country to introduce legislation to curb the nation's intake of sugar. Many of us drink a can of soft drink a day. But did you know that there are about 9 teaspoons of sugar in a can? I'm not talking about simply cutting sugar out of your tea or coffee. That is a bare minimum requirement. Let's talk a little about sugar.

WHAT IS SUGAR?
There are a number of different sugars, but the one you buy in bags is known chemically as sucrose. Sucrose is a molecule created by two simpler sugars, fructose and glucose, joined together. Natural sweeteners such as honey, agave nectar and maple syrup contain one or all of them. Even fruit contains them, albeit in lower concentrations (even beans, vegetables and grains have a little). Irrespective of their source, the body processes sugars the same way for use as energy, but what it needs is a slow, steady supply rather than a series of deluges.

Even if you think that you don't need to worry about sugar because you don't have a sweet tooth, think again. Products such as soup, tomato ketchup, fruit juices and salad dressings can contain as much, and often more sugar, than cakes, pastries, cookies and biscuits. The organization Action on Sugar suggests swapping cakes or biscuits for an alternative with less sugar, such as a currant bun or scone. The other sugar trap is alcohol. Diet mixers are a good substitute with spirits, but don't forget that a glass of wine, cider or beer may also contain sugar.

In recent years, some manufacturers have begun to reduce the added sugar in some products often by substituting artificial sweeteners. Many smaller producers are bringing healthier options to the fore. Products are sweetened with fruit or alternative sweeteners, such as xylitol. Meanwhile, there is a growing appetite for fresh sugar-free cakes. And while food packaging labels contain details of sugar content, it's important to remember that they don't differentiate between naturally occurring sugars, in fruit, vegetables and unsweetened dairy products, all of which are considered acceptable, and added sugars.

Added sugars to watch out for include cane and beet sugar, honey, any kind of syrup, dextrose, sucrose, fructose, glucose, maltose, molasses, hydrolyzed starch or invert sugar. Some foods have color-coded panels that give traffic-light indicators of sugar levels, but these only work as a rough guide.

WHAT TO DO
So, what should you do? The best approach is to re-train your palate to reduce its craving for the super-sweet with simple steps. At breakfast time you could try replacing marmalade or jam on your toast with sliced banana, low-fat cream cheese or eggs. You could also swap those lethal sugar-packed cereals for wholegrain versions. Although these are small steps, but they are in the right direction. The bottom line is that sugar is the new cancer. You have to cut it out. Read the labels on every food you buy and you'll be shocked on just how much sugar they contain.

References:

[1] *Carbohydrates and Health*

RULE #12. STOP EATING WHITE BREAD

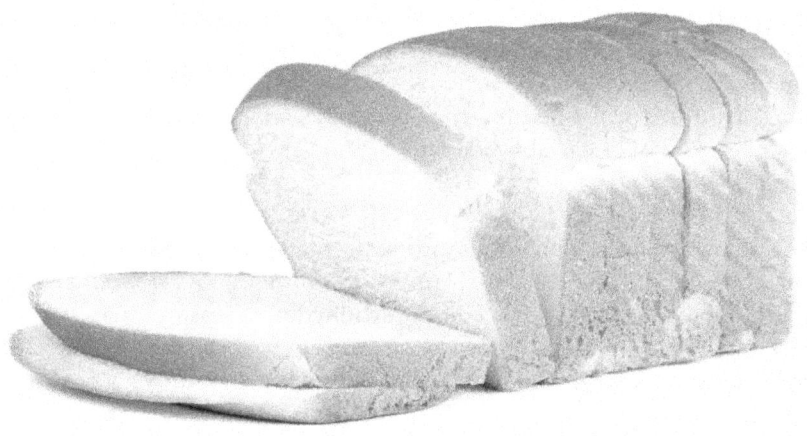

Believe it or not white bread is not good for your health. This may surprise many people, particularly British and Irish people who often start the day with toasted white bread and would have a sandwich at lunchtime. Stop eating it. If you want to improve your health, lose some weight and avoid the possibility of ending up with type II diabetes, then stay away from white bread by which I mean exclude it completely from your diet. Why do I say this? Let me tell you a little about how white bread is made.

HOW WHITE BREAD IS MADE

White bread is made from refined white flour. This flour is made up of several unwholesome constituents and very little in the way of nutrients and dietary fiber which is vital for a healthy digestive system and a stable metabolism. Refined white flour is produced from the whole wheat grain. It is then subjected to the refining process. This removes all traces of the husk, or bran and along with it all the goodness contained in the grain. Next it is bleached using chemical bleaching agents. These agents contain chlorine and are dried in kilns at high temperature to kill any remaining beneficial constituents.

What is left is an insipid, bland, tasteless powder to which the bakers add gluten. Gluten is a product to which an increasing number of consumers are becoming allergic. The only reason gluten is added is to help produce a more evenly risen and air filled loaf.

The bakers will also add sugar and salt both of which will enhance the taste of the bread. But sugar is also added to enable the baker's yeast to prove the dough and make it rise. Salt is added to check the progress of the yeast and prevent the loaf from rising too much, or over-proving. If you eat the average supermarket's own brand cheapest white bread you might as well be eating cardboard, in terms its blandness and lack of any useful dietary benefit whatsoever. While artisan small bakery bread and home-made loaves will taste better because they are made using refined white flour they are still devoid of any health benefits.

WHY WHITE BREAD IS BAD FOR YOU

As with white pasta and other products made from refined white flour, white bread contains a large proportion of high GI carbohydrates. GI stands for glycemic index. These carbohydrates ensure that sugars are quickly released into the bloodstream causing a sharp rise in blood sugar levels. This rise triggers a similarly rapid release of the body's own sugar regulating hormone, insulin. Insulin is secreted in the pancreas and is responsible for regulating blood sugar levels.

Insulin is what people suffering with diabetes need to inject to regulate their blood sugar levels because their body does not produce sufficient naturally. As you are probably aware type II diabetes is a rapidly spreading disease brought on by too frequent imbalances in blood sugar levels causing insulin production to become overworked. This eventually leads to the problem and all the negative health aspects associated with it.

Other negative health aspects associated with it include raised levels of bad LDL cholesterol in your bloodstream. This can cause heart disease including the narrowing of the arteries. When levels of LDL cholesterol become too high, artery walls thicken. This causes blockages which, in turn, can cause high blood pressure and thrombosis otherwise known as blood clots. Another negative aspect of eating white bread is its effect of slowing down the body's metabolism. This reduces the efficiency of our digestive system, causing our body to store greater amounts of fat, the type of fat that usually accumulates around the midriff.

In fact, this is one of the main reasons why weight loss is so difficult for people who continue to eat white bread. One study even shows that white bread causes weight gain. The study [1] published in *BMC Health* in October 2014 involved 9,267 Spanish university graduates for a mean period of 5 years. The results showed that eating two slices (120 grams) of white bread per day was linked to a 40% greater risk of weight gain and obesity.

Not only does white bread make you gain weight but it also makes you feel more sluggish, lethargic and less inclined to want to exercise. The lack of dietary fiber is a big problem for your digestible tract, especially the intestines that complete digestion and facilitates waste in leaving the body. When there is little or no dietary fiber present in your diet, your colon will suffer and be unable to effectively remove all waste products from your body. This can cause complications and illnesses like Crohn's Disease, Irritable Bowel Syndrome (IBS) and can result in colon cancer.

ALTERNATIVES TO REGULAR WHITE BREAD
Fortunately, there are many healthy alternatives to conventional wheat bread. You don't have to give up bread from your diet, just white bread. The viable alternative is of course brown bread, otherwise known as wholemeal or wholegrain bread. Brown bread is produced from wholemeal flour which is not refined in the same way as white flour.

Wholemeal flour retains the husk of the wheat, or bran which is where all the nutrients and dietary fiber exist. Furthermore, there is no bleaching and gluten levels are usually lower than in white bread. Wholemeal flour contains much lower levels of high GI carbohydrates than white flour and also higher levels of low GI carbohydrates. The low ones work in the opposite way to high GI carbohydrates, as the low ones which are in wholemeal bread produce the slow release of sugars into the bloodstream.

The result of this is that insulin is only slowly released into the bloodstream and in far lower amounts. Rather than being inhibited, the metabolism is stimulated. This means that your digestive system benefits from a boost in efficiency and less fat gets stored. This is great news for those of us looking to reduce our body-weight. Wholemeal flour products like brown bread contain high levels of dietary fiber. This is essential for the functioning of the colon and the complete digestion of food and waste elimination.

They also contain lower levels of bad LDL cholesterol with higher levels of good HDL cholesterol resulting in healthy arteries and a more normal blood pressure. Finally, brown bread actually tastes better and doesn't have that cloying, pasty texture that massed produced white bread have.

EZEKIEL

There are other alternatives as well, one of which is Ezekiel bread. Although not very well know Ezekiel bread is probably the healthiest bread on the market. What is it? While the majority of bread contains added sugar, Ezekiel bread contains none. It is also made from organic, sprouted whole grains. The sprouting process changes the nutrient composition of the grains significantly.

Unlike the majority of commercially produced breads, which consist primarily of refined wheat or pulverized whole wheat, Ezekiel bread contains several different types of grains and legumes. For example, it contains four types of cereal grains: Wheat, Millet, Barley and Spelt and two types types of legumes: Soybeans and Lentils. All the grains and all the legumes are organically grown and allowed to sprout before they are processed, mixed together and baked to produce the final product.

However, it is important to note that wheat, barley and spelt all contain gluten, so Ezekiel bread is a no-no for anyone who suffers with celiac disease or gluten sensitivity. However, keep in mind that all wheat breads do contain gluten. Some other options include oopsie bread, cornbread and almond flour bread. But the bottom line is that if you want to lose weight stop eating white bread.

References:

[1] *Glycemic load, glycemic index, bread and incidence of overweight/obesity in a Mediterranean cohort: the SUN project.*

5 WHAT NOT TO DRINK

RULE #13. DITCH SOFT DRINKS AND FRUIT JUICES

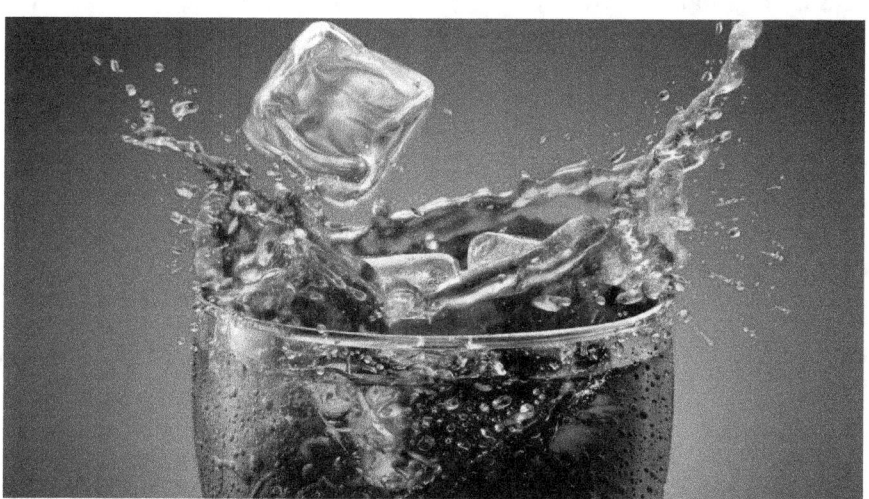

Recently, a client told me that they had given up drinking *Coca Cola* with their meals and snack and switched to the "healthier" option of fruit juices. I asked her what kind of fruit juice and she said: "Just fruit juice. Not from concentrate. Now, I've got one of my five a day." Big mistake. Big, big mistake. If you are trying to lose weight stop drinking sodas, soft drinks and fruit juices.

But I hear you say: "Aren't fruit juices healthier than say drinking a can of Coke?" That ain't necessarily so. Always read the label, carefully. Just because it says "fruit" doesn't actually mean real fruit. In certain cases, fruit juice can be worse for you than your average soft drink. The reality is that manufacturers do not always tell the truth. Some will try and trick you into believing that the product you are buying is healthy when in actual fact it isn't. For example, sometimes "fruit juice" isn't actually made with real fruit at all, it is just fruit flavored sugar water. There may not even be any actual fruit in there. It might, and often does, just contain water, sugar and some chemicals that taste like fruit.

If you see "100% fruit juice" on the label you should still avoid it. Why? Because the problem with fruit juice, is that it's like fruit except that all the healthy benefits have been extracted. But, don't whole fruits contain sugar? Yes, they do. Whole fruits contain some sugar, but that sugar is bound within the fibrous cell walls, which slows down the release of the sugar into the bloodstream. The difference with fruit juice is there is no fiber, there is no chewing resistance and consequently nothing to prevent you from consuming massive amounts of sugar within a very short period of time. This is not good.

Remember, one cup of orange juice contains almost as much sugar as two whole oranges. One study [1] published in the respected medical journal *The Lancet* in June 2014 shows that the sugar content of fruit juice is actually very similar to sugar-sweetened beverages like *Coca Cola*. The packaging may actually claim that the drink has something like "added vitamins and nutrients." However, the small amounts of vitamins and antioxidants in the juice do not make up for the large amount of sugar.

I've even picked up fruit juice in my local supermarket which is labelled "Pure Fruit Juice – 100%. What does this mean? What it means is that unless it was squeezed from oranges there and then in the store it's probably very old. The manufacturing process works like this: after being squeezed from the fruit, the juice is usually stored in massive oxygen-depleted holding tanks for up to a year before it is packaged. Bet you didn't know that. Obviously, this present problems.

The main problem with this method is that it tends to remove most of the flavor from the oranges. But the manufacturers have a cunning plan. They add so-called "flavor packs" to the juice, to bring back the flavor that was lost during processing. So, even if you're buying the highest quality juices at the supermarket, the likelihood is that they are still far from their original state. That's the expensive fruit juice.

Some of the lowest quality ones don't even resemble fresh-squeezed fruit juice at all. One I picked up in my supermarket yesterday contained 28% sugar! Basically, these are just fruit-flavored sugar water.

Manufacturers will argue that fruit juice contains vitamins, minerals and antioxidants. So what? Big deal. It also lacks fiber and is overloaded with sugar. Fruit juice is missing most of the benefits that makes whole fruit healthy. For example, orange juice does contain vitamin C and is a decent source of folate, potassium and vitamin B1 and two studies have shown that it also contains antioxidants, some of which can increase the antioxidant value of the blood.

But, my friends, calorie for calorie, or sugar gram for sugar gram, it is nutritionally poor compared to whole oranges and other plant foods like vegetables. This was the finding in a study [2] published in the October 2013 edition of the *Journal Academy of Nutrition and Dietetics*.

Still not convinced? Then take a look at the breakdown for a 12 ounce (350 ml) portion of *Coca Cola* compared to apple juice. *Coca Cola* contains 140 calories and 40 grams of sugar. That's 10 teaspoons of sugar. Apple juice contains 165 calories and 39 grams of sugar which comprises 9.8 teaspoons. What's the difference? Well, 0.2 of course but you know know what I mean.

When we eat a whole orange it takes some not inconsiderable effort to chew and swallow it. The sugar in the orange is also bound within fibrous structures that breaks down slowly during digestion. Not only that, but fruit is also very filling. It's hard to eat more than two pieces of whole fruit at the one sitting.

Because of this, the sugar in whole fruit makes its way to the liver slowly and in small amounts. The liver can easily metabolize these small amounts without being overloaded. But this is not the case when you drink orange juice. If you drink a large glass of orange or any other fruit juice, it is the equivalent of consuming several pieces of fruit in a very short amount of time, except there is no fiber in it.

What happens is that the large amount of sugar gets absorbed and travels to the liver very quickly, just like when you drink a sugar-sweetened beverage. A large part of the sugar found in fruit juice is fructose. Studies have shown that the liver is the only organ that can metabolize fructose in meaningful amounts. So, what happens when the liver takes in more fructose than it can handle? Some of it gets turned into fat.

Five separate studies have shown that some of the fat can lodge in the liver and contribute to fat buildup and insulin resistance. Although small amounts of fruit juice or soda are unlikely to cause major problems for healthy, lean and active people, this is not the case for those who are overweight. Studies published in the *American Journal of Clinical Nutrition* and the *Physiological Review* show that for those who are overweight or have diet-related metabolic problems this is a disaster.

Controlled metabolic studies show that liquid sugar can cause insulin resistance, raise triglycerides and small, dense LDL cholesterol, elevate oxidized LDL cholesterol and cause belly fat accumulation in as little as 10 weeks. Although most of the studies are using sugar-sweetened or fructose-sweetened drinks, there is no evidence to suggest that 100% fruit juice would be any different. The sugar molecules are identical and your liver is unable to differentiate.

A study showed that 480 ml (16 ounces) of grape juice per day for 3 months caused insulin resistance and increased waist circumference in overweight individuals. Another study [3], published in 2010 in the journal *JAMA* showed that consuming two or more servings of fruit juice per day was associated with more than a doubled risk of gout in women.

Now, I want to talk about the dangers of liquid calories. Let's begin by dispelling some myths. Firstly, not all calories are the same. By this I mean that different foods go through different metabolic pathways and have different effects on hunger, hormones and the brain centers that control body weight.

One of the functions of the brain is to regulate energy balance. When you add a food to your diet, your brain compensates by making you eat less of other foods instead. For example, if we were to start eating two boiled potatoes every day, we would subconsciously end up eating less of other foods, so our total calorie intake wouldn't increase much, if at all.

However, liquid calories don't work the same way as calories from solid foods. When you add liquid calories to your diet, like for example, apple juice, they don't compensate by eating less of other foods instead.

This is one of the reasons that sugary drinks are among the most fattening foods you can take. They don't contribute to fullness, so overall we take in more calories.

One study in children [4] published in *The Lancet* in February 2001 showed that the risk of obesity was increased by 60% for each daily serving of sugar-sweetened beverages.

There is no evidence to suggest that fruit juices would have a different effect than sugary drinks, if they are consumed in the same amounts. In fact, several studies show that fruit juice is linked to an increased risk of obesity and type II diabetes, while whole fruit is linked to a decreased risk.

Overall, drinking fruit juice in small amounts may be acceptable for certain correct weighted individuals, but it is important to remember that the reality is that fruit juice is very similar to sugar filled soft drinks. Your liver can't tell the difference. So, the bottom line is to stay away from all soft drinks and fruit juices and drink water instead.

References:

[1] *Fruit juice: just another sugary drink?*

[2] *Deconstructing a fruit serving: comparing the antioxidant density of select whole fruit and 100% fruit juices.*

[3] *Fructose-Rich Beverages and the Risk of Gout in Women*

[4] *Relation between consumption of sugar-sweetened drinks and childhood obesity*

RULE #14. MODERATE YOUR ALCOHOL INTAKE

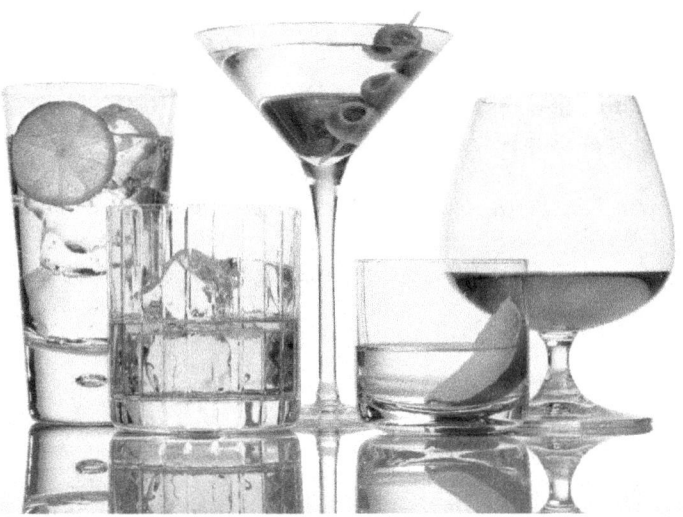

Alcohol and weight loss don't mix. However, you can still enjoy a healthy lifestyle and take an occasional drink. In fact, many experts note the potential health benefits of consuming a single drink per day, including a reduced risk for high blood pressure. The problem is that if you are exceeding one drink daily, you might be sabotaging your weight loss plans. I'm not going to lecture anyone about the dangers of alcohol. My sister was an alcoholic. Five of my uncles were also alcoholics. My two best friends are alcoholics and up until recently I used to drink one bottle of wine a day. As a result I suffer from very high blood pressure and moderate heart problems. Let's discuss first of all how alcohol works in your system.

HOW ALCOHOL WORKS IN YOUR SYSTEM

Alcohol is metabolized differently than other foods and beverages. Normally, your body gets its energy from the calories in carbs, fats and proteins, which are slowly digested and absorbed within the gastrointestinal system. However, this digestive process changes when you imbibe alcohol. When you start drinking the alcohol in your system attracts immediate attention and requires no digestion. Why does it attract immediate attention. Because your body treats it like a toxin, which, let's fact it, it is.

On an empty stomach, the alcohol molecules diffuse through the stomach wall quickly and can reach the brain and liver in a matter of minutes. The process is slower when you have food in your system. However, as soon as that food enters the small intestine, the alcohol is given first priority and is absorbed quickly into the bloodstream.

As the alcohol reaches the liver for processing, the liver gives the alcohol its undivided attention. If you drink very slowly, all the alcohol is collected by the liver and processed immediately, thus avoiding all other body systems. If you drink quickly, the liver cannot keep up with the processing needs. The alcohol then continues to circulate in the body until the liver is available to process it.

When the body is focused on processing alcohol, it cannot properly break down foods containing carbohydrates and fat. Therefore, these calories are converted into body fat and are carried away for permanent storage in your body. You should also know that alcohol is a diuretic. That means is causes water loss and dehydration. Along with this water loss you lose important minerals, such as magnesium, potassium, calcium and zinc.

The problem is that these minerals are crucial to the maintenance of fluid balance, chemical reactions, and muscle contraction and relaxation. Generally speaking, alcohol contains 7 calories per gram and offers no nutritional value. In fact, all it does is add empty calories to your diet. I'm not saying you shouldn't drink alcohol. I'm saying you should limit it to one drink per day if you really want to lose weight.

THE BAD THINGS ABOUT ALCOHOL

You have probably read media reports that alcohol is actually good for you. A small amount like one glass per day probably is. However, let's not kid ourselves. Alcohol affects our body in negative ways. Drinking alcohol may help induce sleep, but the sleep you get isn't very deep. As a result, you get less rest. This can result in you eating more calories the following day. Also, alcohol can increase the amount of acid that your stomach produces, causing your stomach lining to become inflamed. Over time, excessive alcohol use can lead to serious health problems, including high blood pressure, stomach ulcers, liver disease, and heart troubles.

Furthermore, alcohol lowers your inhibitions, which is detrimental to your diet plans. In fact, alcohol stimulates your appetite. While you might be full from a comparable amount of calories from food, several drinks might not fill you up.

In addition, studies show that if you drink before or during a meal, both your inhibitions and willpower are reduced. In this state, the chances are that you are more likely to overeat. One way to avoid this is not to drink alcohol until you've finished your meal or to drink a glass of water between alcoholic drinks.

DRINKING INSTEAD OF EATING

Some people think the way around adding calories is to skip a meal to save your calories for drinks later on. This is a bad idea. If you come to the bar hungry, you are even more likely to munch on the snacks. If you plan to drink alcohol in the evening have a healthy meal first. The reason is that you will feel fuller, which will stop you from over indulging on alcohol. If you are worried about a drinks night out try an extra 30 minutes of exercise before you go. This can help balance your calories. At least it's preferable to skipping a meal.

You might think that drinking spirits is more diet-friendly because they have no carbohydrates, while both wine and beer contain carbs. But dieters need to watch calories, and spirits only contain a few calories less than beer or wine. In addition, spirits are often mixed with other drinks, adding even more empty calories. Hard spirits contains around 100 calories per shot, so adding a mixer increases calories even more. If you are going to mix spirits with anything, go for a diet or club soda, instead of fruit juice or regular soda.

Sweeter drinks, whether spirit or wine, tend to have more sugar, and therefore more calories. In that respect, dry wines usually have fewer calories than sweet wines.

The following list below breaks down the number of calories in typical alcoholic drinks: 5 oz of red or white wine have 100 calories; champagne 130; 12 oz of beer have 105 calories for light beer, 140 for regular beer and 170 for dark beer; and an 8 oz gin and tonic has 175 calories while a rum and soda has 180.

IS ALCOHOL GOOD FOR YOUR HEART?
It's complicated. While moderate drinking may offer health benefits, drinking more than one glass a day can cause a number of health problems.

In several studies of diverse populations, moderate alcohol consumption has been associated with a reduced risk for certain cardiovascular diseases, such as coronary heart disease. But it should be remembered that these studies were observational, not experimental. Accordingly, the results have some limitations.

The first major study was in 1999 when a meta-analysis was conducted on all experimental studies to date to assess the effects of moderate alcohol intake on various health measures (such as HDL "good" cholesterol levels and triglycerides), and other biological markers associated with risk of coronary heart disease. Later, researchers conducted a systematic review of 63 studies that examined adults without known cardiovascular disease before and after alcohol use.

The results of the study [1] were published in the 2011 of the *British Medical Journal*. The analysis of these numerous studies suggested that moderate alcohol consumption helps to protect against heart disease in several ways.

It listed those ways as raising HDL "good" cholesterol; increasing apolipoprotein A1, a protein that has a specific role in lipid (fat) metabolism and is a major component of HDL "good" cholesterol; decreasing fibrinogen, a soluble plasma glycoprotein that is a part of blood clot formation; lowering blood pressure; reducing plaque accumulation in the arteries; and, decreasing the clumping of platelets and the formation of blood clots.

However, the studies did not demonstrate any relationship between moderate alcohol intake and total cholesterol level or LDL "bad" cholesterol. And while some studies associated alcohol intake to increased triglycerides, the most recent analysis of moderate alcohol intake in healthy adults showed no such relationship.

WHAT IS MODERATE DRINKING?
A moderate alcohol intake is defined as up to one drink per day for women and up to two drinks per day for men. One drink contains 0.6 fluid ounces of alcohol and is defined as: 12 fl. oz. of regular beer (5% alcohol); 4-5 fl. oz. of wine (12% alcohol); 1.5 fl. oz. of 80-proof distilled spirits (40% alcohol) and 1 fl. oz. of 100-proof distilled spirits (50% alcohol).

ARE SOME TYPES OF ALCOHOL BETTER THAN OTHERS?

The results are inconclusive. While a few research studies suggest that wine maybe more beneficial than beer or sprits in the prevention of heart disease, most studies do not support an association between type of alcoholic beverage and the prevention of heart disease. At the moment there is no hard evidence that drinking wine for its antioxidant content will prevent heart disease. And it still remains uncertain whether red wine offers any heart-protecting advantage over white wine or other types of alcoholic beverages.

HEALTH RISK OF BINGE OR HEAVY DRINKING

Whatever about moderate drinking having some health benefits, the fact is that heavy or binge drinking can have a toxic effect on your health and your heart. You are considered a heavy drinker if you consume more than three drinks on any day or more than seven drinks per week for women and more than four drinks on any day or more than fourteen drinks per week for men.

Heavy drinking in particular can damage the heart and lead to high blood pressure, alcoholic cardiomyopathy (enlarged and weakened heart), congestive heart failure, and stroke. When you drink heavily you allow more fat into the circulation in your body which raises your triglyceride level. Heavy drinking is also associated with an increased risk of cirrhosis of the liver, cancer of the gastrointestinal tract and colon and breast cancer.

Binge drinking is the consumption within two hours of four or more drinks for women and five or more drinks for men.

PEOPLE WHO SHOULD NOT DRINK ALCOHOL AT ALL

According to the 2010 Dietary Guidelines for Americans, there are certain people should not drink alcohol at all. They include adults who cannot restrict their alcohol drinking to moderate levels; women who are pregnant or may become pregnant; anyone taking a medication (prescription or over-the counter) that can interact with alcohol; people with certain medical conditions such as liver disease, hypertriglyceridemia, and pancreatitis; and those who plan to drive, operate machinery or take part in other activities that require attention, skill, or coordination or in situations where impaired judgment could cause injury or death, such as swimming.

I'M GOING TO DRINK ANYWAY SO WHAT'S THE BEST DRINK FOR WEIGHT LOSS

OK, so you want to lose weight but you don't want to give up alcohol. I hear you. Even if you are careful about your alcohol consumption, all drinks are not created equal on the dieting scale which means that some choices are better than others. The best drinks for this purpose are red and white wine, Scotch, vodka and light beer, all of which contain about 100 calories.

Wine is the most calorie friendly choice with a typical 20 calories per ounce. Spirits are higher in calories per ounce than wine, and as they are often mixed with soda, increases the calorie count. If you're going to drink spirits, use calorie-free mixers like diet soda or diet tonic water.

Once you start mixing spirits with juice and other sweeteners to create cocktails, both calories and carbs can go up significantly. For example, a Pina Colada has 250 calories, a Margarita 150 and a Cosmopolitan 215. Beer is the next best choice for dieters with, about 150 calories per 12-ounce serving. Choosing light beers will drop your caloric intake without sacrificing much flavor. For example, a light beer will contain 108 calories per glass while a lager contains 170 and an ale 220.

The bottom line is that if you are trying to lose weight any type of alcohol is a no-no. But if, like me, you can resist anything but temptation, one drink for a female and two for a male are the maximum daily drinks you should take.

References:

[1] *Effect of alcohol consumption on biological markers associated with risk of coronary heart disease.*

RULE #15. DO MORE DAIRY

LOW CARB FOOD PYRAMID

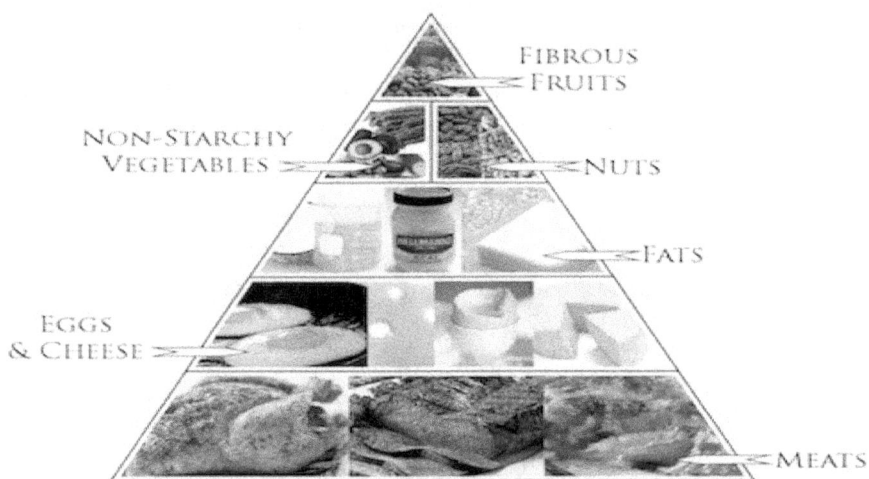

Many studies have shown that low-carb diets are very effective for weight loss. But, in the past, many experts stated that increased fat in the diet is a leading cause of health problems in general and heart disease in particular.

In fact, this is the current position held by the majority of mainstream health organizations. They generally recommend that people restrict dietary fat to less than 30% of total calories. In effect, this amounts to a low-fat diet. However, in the last decade, an increasing number of studies have caused doubt on and directly challenged the low-fat dietary approach.

Many health professionals now believe that a low-carb diet which is higher in fat and protein is a much better option to treat obesity and other chronic diseases. This evidence is based on over twenty recent studies which compared low-carb and low-fat diets. All of these studies were randomized controlled trials, the gold standard of science and all are published in respected, peer-reviewed journals.

The majority of studies achieved statistically significant differences in weight loss (always in favor of low-carb). There are six results which are worth noting. Firstly, the low-carb groups often lost 2-3 times as much weight as the low-fat groups. In a few instances there was no significant difference. Secondly, in most cases, calories were restricted in the low-fat groups, while the low-carb groups could eat as much as they wanted.

Thirdly, when both groups restricted calories, the low-carb dieters still lost more weight, (although in fairness it was not always significant). Fourthly, there was only one study where the low-fat group lost more weight although the difference was small (0.5 kg – 1.1 lb) and not statistically significant. Fifthly, in several of the studies, weight loss was greatest in the beginning. Then people started regaining the weight over time as they abandoned the diet. And, finally, when the researchers looked at abdominal fat directly, which is the unhealthy visceral fat, low-carb diets were well in front.

WHAT ABOUT LDL CHOLESTEROL?
Despite the concerns expressed by many, low-carb diets generally do not raise Total and LDL cholesterol levels on average. Low-fat diets do lower Total and LDL cholesterol, but it is usually only temporary. After 6 to 12 months, the difference is not statistically significant.

There have been some anecdotal reports by doctors who treat patients with low-carb diets, that they can lead to increases in LDL cholesterol and some advanced lipid markers for a small percentage of individuals. However, none of the above studies noted any of these adverse effects. The few studies that looked at advanced lipid markers only showed improvements.

WHAT ABOUT HDL CHOLESTEROL?
One of the best ways to raise HDL cholesterol levels is to eat more fat. For this reason, it is not surprising to see that low-carb diets (higher in fat) raise HDL significantly more than low-fat diets. Having higher HDL levels is correlated with improved metabolic health and a lower risk of cardiovascular disease. Having low HDL levels is one of the key symptoms of the metabolic syndrome. The majority of these studies (18 of the 23) recorded changes in HDL cholesterol levels.

WHAT ABOUT BLOOD PRESSURE?

When measured, blood pressure tended to decrease on both low-carb and low-fat diets.

WERE THERE ANY ADVERSE EFFECTS?

Despite the concerns expressed by many health experts in the past, there were absolutely no reports of serious adverse effects that were attributable to either diet. Overall, the low-carb diet was well tolerated and had an outstanding safety profile.

These studies are scientific evidence, as good as it gets, that low-carb is much more effective than the low-fat diet that is still being recommended all over the world.

THE BOTTOM LINE

The bottom line is that limiting carbs and eating more fat and protein reduces your appetite and helps you eat fewer calories. This can result in weight loss that is up to three times greater than that from a standard low-fat diet.

A low-carb diet can also improve many risk factors for disease. So, my advice is to start eating non-fat and low-fat yogurt (but watch the sugar content!) and cheese. Research shows that you get the best results from dairy products themselves and not fortified foods. Aim for 1,200 mg which includes about three servings a day.

5 THINGS TO DO TO LOSE WEIGHT

RULE #16. START MINDFUL EATING

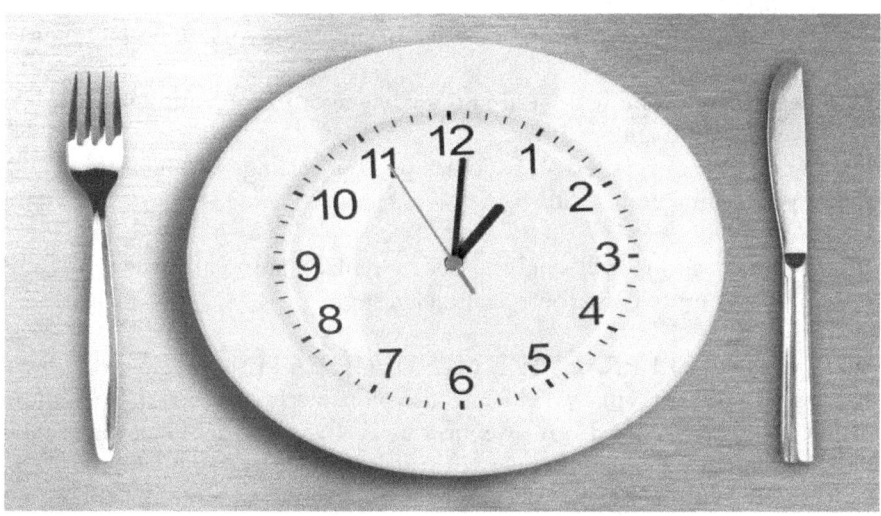

Mindful eating is a particular type of eating technique that can assist you in controlling your eating habits. Evidence suggest that it can effect weight loss, reduce binge eating and generally help you feel better. The term comes from the Buddhist concept of mindfulness.

Irish psychotherapist Padraig O'Morain describes mindfulness in the following terms: "At its simplest, mindfulness means being aware of what you are doing while you are doing it. This means being aware that you are breathing, walking, driving, running making a phone call, cooking a meal and so on. When you have thoughts, notice that you have thoughts and come back to awareness of what you are actually doing. When you are emotional just notice the emotion – not trying to deepen it and not trying to push it away – and come back to awareness of what you are doing."

In effect, mindfulness is a form of meditation that helps you recognize and cope with your emotions and physical sensations. It has been useful in treating several conditions such as depression, anxiety, eating disorders, and other food-related behaviors. You could say that mindful eating is about using mindfulness to reach a state of full attention to your experiences, cravings and physical cues while you are eating. So what exactly does mindful eating involve?

- It involves eating slowly and without distraction.
- Listening to physical hunger cues.
- Eating only until you're full.
- Distinguishing between actual hunger and non-hunger triggers for eating.
- Engaging your senses to be aware of smells, colors, sounds, textures and tastes.
- Learning to cope with guilt and anxiety about food eating to maintain overall health and well-being.
- Being aware of the effect food has on your feelings and figure
- Appreciating your food.

All of these actions will enable you to replace automatic thoughts and reactions with more conscious, healthier responses.

WHY SHOULD I PRACTICE MINDFUL EATING?

In today's fast moving world we are constantly distracted and these distractions have shifted our attention away from the actual act of eating and enjoying our food. How many of us eat while engaging in conversation, watching television, driving, playing games on our computers or talking on our cell phones? Often, we don't even look at the food we are eating. Sometimes we just scoff our food down without even thinking about what we are eating.

In truth, for most of us, eating has become a mindless act. This is not good, particularly when you consider that it can take our brains up to half an hour to realize we are full. If we eat too fast, then we end up eating more than we actually need.

This is a very common factor in binge eating. But if we eat mindfully we can restore our attention to our food and eating and actually slow down, which makes eating an intentional act rather than an automatic one.

By increasing our recognition of physical hunger and fullness cues, two things happen. Firstly, we are better able to distinguish between emotional and actual, physical hunger. Secondly, we increase our awareness of triggers that make us want to eat in circumstances where we're not actually hungry. Once we can identify these triggers we can create a space between them and the response. This allows us the time and freedom to actually choose our response.

WEIGHT LOSS PROGRAMS

In my opinion, weight loss programs are not effective in the long term. This opinion is based on the scientific fact that about 85% of obese individuals who lose weight return to or exceed their initial weight within a few years. Four separate studies show that binge eating, emotional eating, external eating and eating in response to food cravings have been linked to weight gain and weight regain after successful weight loss. Chronic exposure to stress may also play a large role in overeating and the development of obesity.

In fact, according to an article [1] in the *Journal of Obesity* in 2011 the vast majority of studies agree that mindful eating helps you lose weight by changing eating behaviors and reducing stress. The study showed that a six week group seminar on mindful eating among obese individuals resulted in an average weight loss of 9 lbs (4 kg) during the seminar and the twelve week follow-up period.

Another six month seminar resulted in an average weight loss of 26 lbs (12 kg), without any regained weight in the following three month period. By changing the way we think about food, we can replace the negative feelings that may be associated with eating with awareness, improved self-control and positive emotions. Once we properly address unwanted eating behaviors we increase the possibility of successful long-term weight loss.

BINGE EATING V MINDFUL EATING

What constitutes binge eating? Bing eating involves eating a large amount of food in a short amount of time, in a manner which is both mindless and without control. Binge eating contributes to eating disorders and serious weight gain. A study [2] published in the *Journal Obstetrics Gynecology Canada* in 2007 showed that almost 70% of binge eaters are obese.

This study was supported by two previous studies published in the journal *Obesity* in June 2007 and *Comprehensive Psychiatry* in March 2007.

So, it may interest you to know that four separate studies have shown that mindful eating drastically reduces the severity and frequency of binge eating. One particular study [3] in the Journal *Health Psychology* in 1999 found that after a six week group intervention in obese women, binge eating episodes decreased from four to one and a half times per week. The severity of each episode also decreased. So there is ample evidence to suggest that not only can mindful eating prevent binge eating but it can also reduce the frequency of binges, as well as the severity of each binge eating episode.

Mindful eating methods have been shown to reduce Emotional eating (eating in response to certain emotions); and External eating (eating in response to environmental food-related cues, such as the sight or smell of food. Unhealthy eating behaviors like these are the most commonly reported problems among obese individuals. Mindful eating provides you with the skills to help you deal with these impulses. It puts you in charge of your responses, instead of you acting on them without thought.

HOW TO PRACTICE MINDFUL EATING

To practice mindfulness, you'll need a series of exercises and meditations. Some find it helpful to attend a seminar, online course or workshop on mindfulness or mindful eating but it is not necessary. The following are some simple ways to get started.

1. DE-STRESS

Studies show that stress, or emotional upheaval, affects levels of the hormone cortisol. In turn, this disrupts both our blood sugar levels and the brain's ability to communicate smoothly with the digestive system. This is why appetite and digestion are so sensitive to our moods. But we can change how our body reacts to food. Begin with a few simple breathing exercises.

Those practicing mindfulness have long known that breathing exercises are a simple way to distract an overactive mind from the other worries of your day. Stress typically makes our breathing shorter and shallower but, by slowing it down and taking deeper breaths, we can reduce stress and boost the oxygenation of the blood which feeds the entire digestive system. Breathing slowly and carefully while eating allows the body to relax. Try using slow, deep belly breaths before you start to eat.

2. CHEW THOROUGHLY

Never underestimate the importance of chewing. Some experts say you should chew each mouthful up to 150 times but this is not really necessary.

Just chew to a pulp. Your mouth is where the digestive process begins. Saliva contains important digestive enzymes which can only begin to work if our food spends a little time in the mouth before being swallowed. Chewing also breaks down food, thus increasing the surface area on which the enzymes can work. This allows the body to receive minerals and nutrients from food and properly utilize its contents.

If we swallow our food too soon then we lose half the digestion process. If whole or poorly-chewed bits of food enter the digestive tract, they can set off a disastrous chain of events. Organs that should be performing necessary functions are called upon to help with digesting.

This causes an inflammatory response, which in turn leads to bloating, wind, acid reflux and heartburn. The majority of bloating comes from wind produced by undigested food. Before you swallow each mouthful, ask yourself if you can chew it any more. If it becomes really tedious, take a few breaths before mouthfuls.

3. EAT SLOWLY
Make every effort to focus on your food and the complete experience of eating. Think about the texture, taste, smell and how the food makes you feel. You can start this process with one meal, or just a snack, and then baby step your way towards more mindful eating from there.

4. ELIMINATE DISTRACTIONS
Stop eating food when you're watching television, surfing the internet, talking on the phone, or even having a conversation. Try and eat in silence because then you are truly aware of what and how much you are eating.

5. DON'T KEEP EATING UNTIL YOU'RE FULL
Never eat until you are full. If you do, then you have eaten too much. Remember a happy stomach needs a little room for your food to mix and properly digest. As I already said, it takes the brain one half hour to realize you are full.

6. DRINK WATER
De-bloat your body by drinking water infused with natural diuretics and detoxifying ingredients. Try adding sliced skinned cucumber and lemon to your water. You can even add cayenne and ginger to jump-start your metabolism. But don't drink water or anything else with meals because the liquid will dilute gastric juices. Instead, avoid water for 30 minutes before meals and wait an hour after before rehydrating. The bottom line is slow down, think about and enjoy what you eat.

References:

[1] *Mindfulness Intervention for Stress Eating to Reduce Cortisol and Abdominal Fat among Overweight and Obese Women: An Exploratory Randomized Controlled Study.*

[2] *Preventing excessive weight gain in adolescents: interpersonal psychotherapy for binge eating.*

[3] *An Exploratory Study of a Meditation-based Intervention for Binge Eating Disorder*

RULE #17. GET YOUR THYROID CHECKED

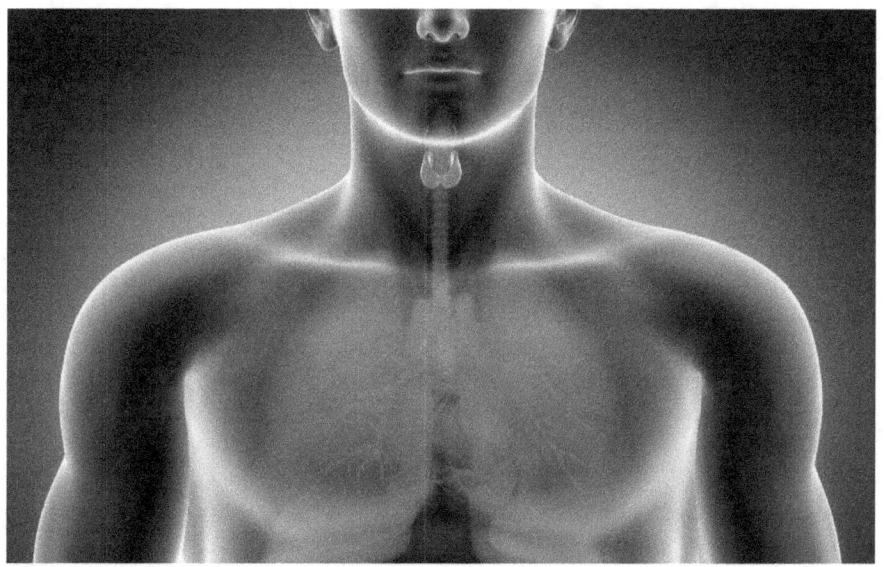

Did you know that according to the Association of Clinical Endocrinologists hypothyroidism or an underactive thyroid gland afflicts 25% of European women. The problem is that many don't even know they are suffering from the condition. The thyroid gland controls your body's metabolism. One of the first signs that it may not be functioning properly is its inability to lose weight. Here's everything you need to know.

WHAT IS THE THYROID GLAND?
The thyroid gland is a butterfly-shaped endocrine gland located in the lower front of the neck. It's function is to make thyroid hormones. These are secreted into the blood and then carried to every tissue in the body. Thyroid

hormone helps the body use energy, stay warm and keep the brain, heart, muscles, and other organs working properly.

WHAT IS THE RELATIONSHIP BETWEEN THYROID, BMR AND WEIGHT?

Differences in BMRs are associated with changes in energy balance. Energy balance reflects the difference between the amount of calories we eat and the amount of calories the body uses. If a high BMR is induced by the administration of drugs, such as amphetamines, studies show that animals often have a negative energy balance which leads to weight loss. Based on these studies researchers have concluded that changes in thyroid hormone levels, which lead to changes in BMR, should also cause changes in energy balance and similar changes in body weight.

However, BMRs are not the whole story relating to weight and thyroid. For example, some studies show that when metabolic rates are reduced by various means like, for example, by decreasing the body temperature, subjects often do not show the expected excess weight gain. Accordingly, the relationship between metabolic rates, energy balance, and weight changes is complex.

There are many other hormones besides thyroid hormone, proteins, and other chemicals that are very important for controlling energy expenditure, food intake, and body weight. As all of these interact on both the brain centers that regulate energy expenditure and tissues throughout the body that control energy expenditure and energy intake, no one can predict with any certainty, the effect of altering only one of these factors (such as thyroid hormone) on body weight as a whole.

Consequently, right now, the American Thyroid Association, are unable to predict the effect of changing thyroid state on any individual's body weight.

But according to Dr. Pamela Peake, the author of *Fight Fat After Forty*, who is professor of Medicine at the University of Maryland, if you feel you have a problem or are suffering from hypothyroidism, your doctor can determine that by a simple blood test. If you are suffering from an underactive thyroid, you'll be treated with a synthetic thyroid supplement, which you will have to take for the rest of your life. This will return your metabolism to normal which should make it easier for you to lose weight.

RULE # 18. DO INTERVAL TRAINING

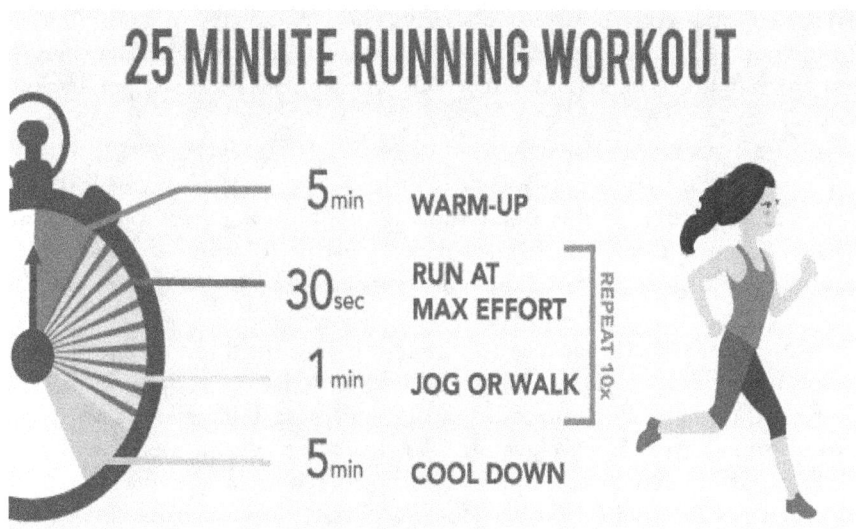

Interval training is a type of training in which you add bursts of high-intensity moves into your workout interspersed with rest or relief periods. According to Dr. Glenn Gaesser, director of the Kinesiology Program at the University of Virginia and author of *The Spark* it is a certain metabolism booster.

A study by researchers at Laval University in Quebec found that high-intensity interval training burns more fat than regular, consistent aerobic exercise.

For example, if you usually jog at a 10-minute-mile pace then add a 30-second sprint every five minutes. Or add a one-minute incline to your treadmill workout every five minutes. Even if you're not a serious exercise head just walk at a normal pace and then add in a 30-second bout of speed-walking every three minutes. It makes a difference. But if you are serious about burning fat read on…

If your aim is to burn fat, you should incorporate interval training into your workout program. As well as being extremely effective to transform your physique, interval training is a great way to hammer out a quick workout. When you incorporate intense periods of work with short recovery segments, interval training helps you give maximum intensity while still maintaining your exercise form.

The best thing about high intensity interval training or HIIT, for short, is that it keeps your body burning fat even after you leave the gym. During a HIIT workout, your body can't shuttle enough oxygen to your muscles during periods of hard work. So, your muscles accumulate a surplus of oxygen that must be repaid after your workout in order to get back to normal.

The result is that your metabolism is revved for hours after you leave the gym. Trainers refer to this phenomena as EPOC or excess post-exercise oxygen consumption. The biggest way to use it to your advantage is to regularly work short, intense bouts of exercise into your workout regimen.

Intense circuits also stimulate muscle-building hormones like growth hormone and IGF-1. This puts your body in a perfect state to build lean mass. And as well as hormone response, interval training also develops the cardiovascular system. By elevating your heart rate during periods of hard work, you'll increase your cardio ability and strengthen your heart. During the short rest intervals, you also increase your recovery capabilities. This means that you are able to recover faster in future workout sessions.

Of course, you don't have to go to a gym to incorporate interval training into your exercise regime. Just follow the principles and do what you can do. You will notice a difference within a week.

RULE #19. IRON UP –PUMP IT, EAT IT

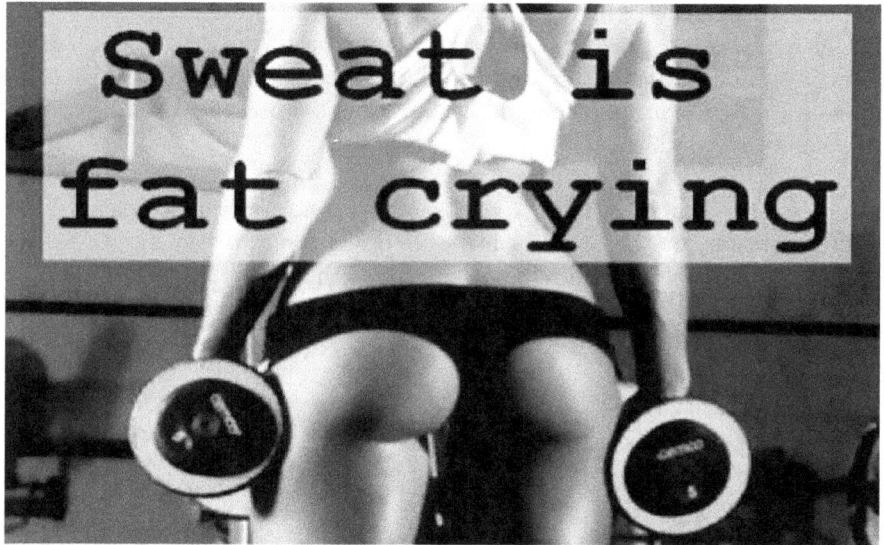

If you are obese and have never undertaken any exercise before then this type of exercise is best left until after you've mastered interval training. The best way to lose weight and maintain loss weight is to begin with baby steps. Do a little of everything in the beginning. Leave the really hard tasks for later on otherwise you will become discouraged. But if exercise is part of you daily or weekly program then pumping iron is something you should definitely do. Weight training is the ultimate way to burn calories fast. Richard Cotton is the chief exercise physiologist for myexerciseplan.com. According to Richard, "a pound of muscle burns up to nine times the calories of a pound of fat."

According to a recent study published in *Medicine and Science in Sport and Exercise* weight training not only increases your resting metabolic rate (the number of calories you burn while sitting on your bum) but it also gives your metabolism an added boost after your exercise is over. It remains working for you for up to two hours after you finish exercising.

Pumping iron is best carried out in a gym and because everyone is different it would be remiss of me to suggest particular exercises. Ask an expert at a gym to devise a simple work-out plan for you and stick with it if it works. Always ask an expert before you start. Otherwise you could easily do yourself some harm.

As well as pumping iron you should also eat iron! If you do not have sufficient iron in your system your body will not be able to get enough oxygen to your cells which will slow down your metabolism. The RDA for adults is around 18 mg and most multivitamins will have this. But you don't need to spend money on multivitamins. You can get an elegant sufficiency of iron through your daily diet. Eat three to four of servings of food which are already rich in iron.

The best foods for iron are spinach, lean red meat, lean pork, chicken, seafood, beans and dried fruits like apricots and raisins. If you are feeling weak or tired all the time there is a possibility that you may be lacking iron. So, visit your doctor and ask them to perform a simple blood test for anemia.

RULE #20. EAT MORE!

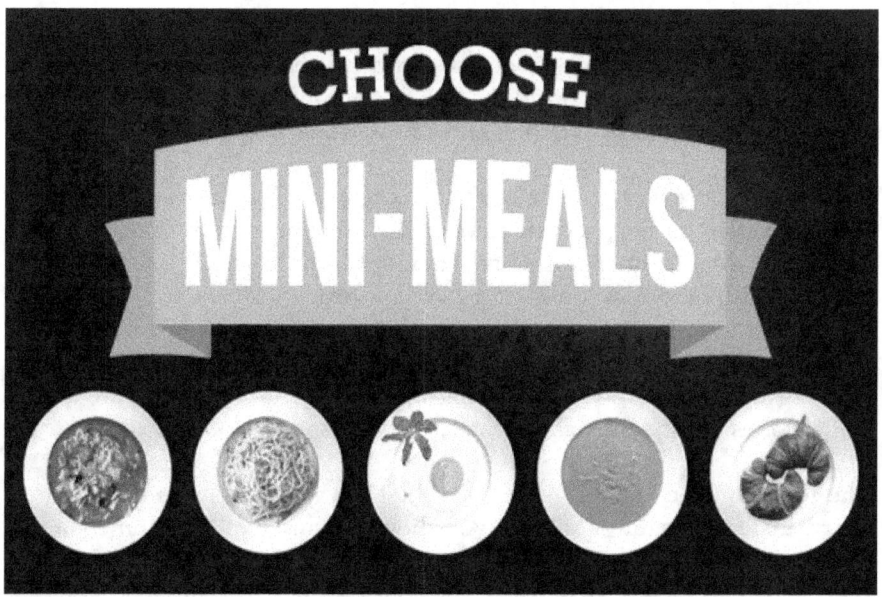

No, that is not a typo. The worst thing you can do when you're trying to lose weight is to skip meals. Some people think that if they skip breakfast or maybe lunch that it will help them lose weight. No, it won't. Do not skip any meal. In fact, rather than eating three substantial meals a day like breakfast, lunch and dinner try and eat six smaller meals a day. Yes, you read that correctly. Eat more often. It's called grazing.

Grazing is the way our bodies were designed to eat. Large and substantial meals tend to burden our digestive system, often causing bloating and lowered energy while the body struggles to digest them. We can prevent this by grazing on smaller meals throughout the day and our body will function more efficiently. When we eat a substantial meal, the sugar level in our blood rises. Once that meal is digested that blood sugar level falls, taking your energy and mood with it. The problem is, the bigger the meal, the bigger the crash. With this comes a greater need for sugary snacks to refuel your body.

But if you eat five or six mini-meals a day, adopting what's called the little-and-often approach your intake of food maintains your energy level stable making it easier for you to cope with everything you have to do in a day. It's not just energy and sugar levels that remain stable. According to the Medical Research Council's Human Nutrition Unit, measurements of fatty acids in the blood also remain stable when you eat little and often.

The little-and-often approach makes it easier to get all the nutrients you need. Generally speaking, those of us who eat three meals a day reply on the same six to seven foodstuffs. But for optimum health, we should be aiming for over a dozen different types of food over two or three days.

Grazers should expect to eat less fat, more carbohydrates and more fruit and vegetables. In fact, several studies show that grazers have higher levels of vitamin C and other nutrients. They also tend to have lower levels of body fat. But, before we go any further, let's make this crystal clear. Grazing is not the same as snacking so if you think you can make one of those six mini-meals a packet of chips or a chocolate bar, forget about it. These are high-fat, high-sugar foods containing little or no nutrients and are loaded with calories which will make you fat. So, what should you eat?

The most important thing is to set yourself what Americans call a calorie salary. Instead of eating "snacks" you should ensure that every time you eat, the food is low in fat and ideally freshly prepared. Think more fruit and vegetables and ensure that whenever you eat carbohydrates you combine them with a little protein because this stabilizes blood sugar further. You may find it difficult to adjust mentally to smaller portions in this split meal approach but it's doable and once you manage you will never go back. If you normally have toast, cereal and fruit for breakfast, have the cereal first, the toast and fruit an hour later.

At lunchtime, eat half your sandwich with a piece of fruit, then have the other half an hour later with some soup or a small salad. In the evening have a smaller dinner than normal and end the day with fruit, a yogurt or a small sandwich an hour later. Trust me, it works.

PART II

FOUR SCIENTIFICALLY PROVEN DIETS THAT WORK

I fully accept, that as well or instead of, adopting my twenty rules on how to permanently lose weight and burn fat some of you may want to undertake a diet as part of of your weight loss program. Having investigated over twenty five popular diet best selling books I believe that the four best diets in the world are as follows:

- The Paleo Diet
- The Mediterranean Diet
- The Low Carb Diet
- The Gluten Free Diet

This belief is based on the evidence of over forty scientific studies that I have examined. What you have to remember is that these diets are not mutually exclusive. You cannot swap parts of one for parts of another. Some of them may actually be contrary to some of the twenty rules you have already read. Finally, none of the diets are written in stone.

This is the problem with diets. No one diet is perfect for everyone. Some diets will suit a particular type of person better than another. Within that "particular type of person" are various different groups. We might have the obese, the overweight, the relatively fit and the fit. We will also have different genders and different types of bodies. The point is that you have to modify each diet to suit your own individual circumstances.

Having read the first part of this book you should now have an understanding of what types of food are generally good for you and what types of foods you should avoid. This remains constant. But some of these diets will ask you to forego foods that I have already recommended. That is not necessarily a contradiction. It just means for that particular diet they want you to do it in their particular way. I've also given you fifteen yummy and delicious recipes for each of these diets. So, enjoy!

THE PALEO DIET

WHAT IS IT?

The paleo diet is based on the types of foods presumed to have been eaten by early humans, our hunter gatherer ancestors, consisting of whole unprocessed food. It is an attempt to emulate the diet of early man who did not suffer from modern day diseases like obesity, diabetes and heart defects. It has been scientifically proven to lead to significant weight loss without the necessity for calorie counting and to improve our general health.

It consists mainly of meat, fish, vegetables, and fruit and excluding dairy or cereal products and processed food. However, in the past number of years, various nutrition based authors have written best selling recipes books adding, subtracting and modifying the diet to suit modern humans, most particularly including bacon and yogurt which kind of defeats the whole purpose of the exercise.

The thing is that paleolithic humans ate different types and varieties of diet depending on where they lived and what was then available. Some ate low-carb diets and some high-carb diets with lots of plants so it is almost impossible to precisely emulate their diet but we can follow the basics in this successful diet.

After all, all we are interested in doing is losing weight and burning fat. So, if the diet or a variation of it works for you, go for it! Here are the basics.

WHAT TO EAT
(Organic if possible)
FISH
Particularly line caught wild fish like salmon, trout, haddock and all types of shellfish.
EGGS
Only eat free range, pastured or omega 3 eggs.
VEGETABLES
All types of fresh vegetables but particularly spinach, broccoli, onions, carrots, tomatoes and potatoes.
FRUIT
Bananas, apples, oranges, pears, avocados, and all types of berries especially blueberries, strawberries and blackberries.
NUTS AND SEEDS
Particularly walnuts, almonds, macadamia nuts, hazelnuts, sunflower seeds, and pumpkin seeds.
MEAT
You can eat meat in moderation like turkey, chicken, pork, beef and lamb.
SPICES
Spices like Himalayan and sea salt, garlic, basil, turmeric, black pepper and rosemary.
HEALTHY FATS
Healthy fats and oils which would include olive oil, lard, coconut, avocado and tallow oil.

WHAT NOT TO EAT
PROCESSED FOODS
This basically means anything made in a factory. Avoid anything that has "low-fat" or "diet" on the label.
SUGARS
All types of sugar and artificial sweeteners and any foods or fruit juices that contain them. This also includes candy, pastries and ice cream.
ALL SOFT DRINKS
Yes, even the Diet and No Sugar varieties
GRAINS
Avoid bread, pasta, rye, barley, spelt and wheat.
DAIRY
Most dairy products especially anything low-fat. (Some versions of this diet allow you to eat butter and cheese)
LEGUMES
Particularly beans and lentils. Some modern diets allow you to eat green beans.

MARGARINE
See trans-fats
VEGETABLE OILS
This includes soybean, sunflower, cotton seed, grapeseed and corn oil.
TRANS-FATS
Trans-fats often referred to as "hydrogenated" or "partially hydrogenated" oils which are found in margarine and various processed foods.

NEW ADDITIONS TO THE PALEO DIET

Recently this diet, more than any other, has evolved to include food which was not available to our ancestors but which modern science has deemed to be good for us. These would include butter, non-processed cheese, quality red wine in moderation, dark chocolate with over 70% cocoa content, quality bacon, black and green tea and black coffee.

SIMPLE MEAL PLANNERS BUT ALSO CHECK THE RECIPES

Most paleo dieticians provide set daily meal plans for breakfast, lunch and dinner and then advise you what you can and cannot eat for snacks. I prefer to stick with my six mini-meals per day to include your snacks. This planner is a template, in other words, switch it around to suit yourself. As regards portions, half a bell pepper, two eggs, one escalope of chicken or pork, two pieces of fruit, salsa made with tomato, cucumber, small tins of fish, cup of olives, berries or a handful of mixed nuts, two mouthfuls of chocolate, and one glass of wine. Drink plenty of water but not with your meal, either before or afterwards.

	SUNDAY
BREAKFAST	Bell Peppers and two Eggs fried in Butter
ELEVEN	Chopped Apple and Pear
LUNCH	Grilled Salmon with Salsa
AFTERNOON	Cup of Nuts or Olives
DINNER	Pork and Red Pepper Stir Fry
NIGHT-TIME	Banana
TREATS	Either glass of Wine or two squares of Chocolate (70%)

	MONDAY
BREAKFAST	Two poached Eggs
ELEVEN	Chopped Apple and Banana
LUNCH	Grilled Pork escalope with Tomato and Cucumber Salsa
AFTERNOON	Cup of Nuts or Olives
DINNER	Small tin of Tuna and warm Boiled Potatoes
NIGHT-TIME	Cup of Cherries
TREATS	Either glass of Wine or two squares of Chocolate (70%)

	TUESDAY
BREAKFAST	Omelette with Vegetables like Peppers, Onions and Tomatoes cooked in Butter
ELEVEN	Chopped Pear and Banana
LUNCH	Burger (no bun) with warm boiled Potatoes or sliced Avocado and Tomato
AFTERNOON	Cup of Nuts or Olives
DINNER	Grilled White Fish and Tomato and Cucumber Salsa
NIGHT-TIME	Two slices of lean Turkey with a chopped Tomato
TREATS	Either glass of Wine or two squares of Chocolate (70%)

	WEDNESDAY
BREAKFAST	Scrambled Eggs
ELEVEN	Chopped Apple and Pear
LUNCH	Grilled Chicken with warm boiled sweet Potatoes
AFTERNOON	Cup of Nuts or Olives
DINNER	Vegetable Stir Fry in olive oil (Peppers, Onion, Spinach, Carrots, Celery etc)
NIGHT-TIME	Banana
TREATS	Either glass of Wine or two squares of Chocolate (70%)

	THURSDAY
BREAKFAST	Two Boiled Eggs
ELEVEN	Chopped Apple and Banana
LUNCH	Small tin of Tuna with Tomato and Cucumber Salsa
AFTERNOON	Cup of Berries
DINNER	Chicken and Bell Peppers Stir Fry in olive oil or Mango, Avocado and Chicken Salad
NIGHT-TIME	Cup of Cherries
TREATS	Either glass of Wine or two squares of Chocolate (70%)

	FRIDAY
BREAKFAST	Sliced Potatoes and Peppers with two Eggs fried in Butter
ELEVEN	Chopped Apple and Pear
LUNCH	Grilled Pork escalope with warm boiled sweet Potatoes
AFTERNOON	Cup of Nuts or Olives
DINNER	Small tin of Tuna with Tomato and Cucumber Salsa
NIGHT-TIME	Banana
TREATS	Either glass of Wine or two squares of Chocolate (70%)

	SATURDAY
BREAKFAST	Vegetable Omelette (Peppers, Onions, Tomatoes etc) cooked in Butter
ELEVEN	Chopped Apple and Banana
LUNCH	Grilled Chicken with Tomato and Cucumber Salsa
AFTERNOON	Cup of Berries
DINNER	Beef and Red and Green Pepper Stir Fry in olive oil
NIGHT-TIME	Cup of Cherries
TREATS	Either glass of Wine or two squares of Chocolate (70%)

15 DELICIOUS PALEO RECIPES

Spicy Seafood Soup

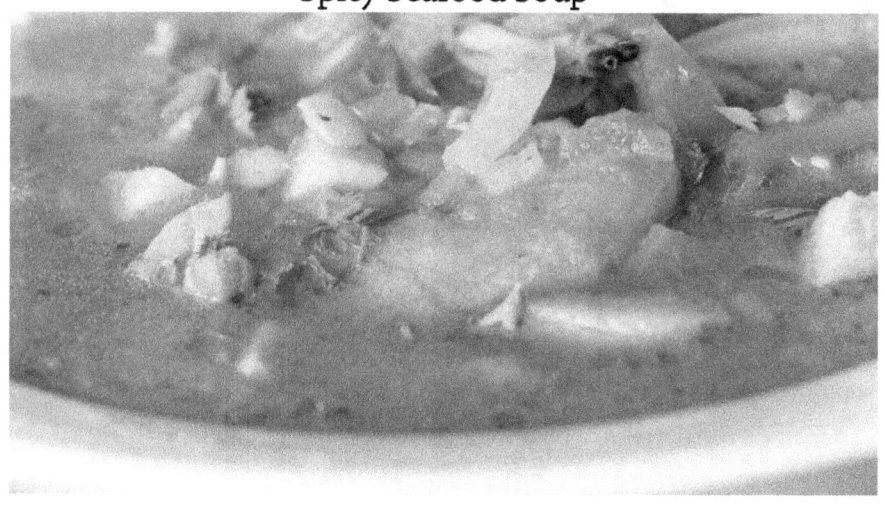

¼ cup lime juice
¼ cup lemon juice
¼ cup chopped coriander (cilantro)
1 portion white cod (cut into four)
1 portion of monkfish (cut into four)
8 raw prawns, peeled and deveined
1 tbsp coconut oil
1 large sliced onion
2 finely diced cloves garlic
4 medium sized plum tomatoes finely diced
1 (14-oz) can full-fat coconut milk

1 ½ tsp of fish sauce
¼ to ½ tsp cayenne pepper
sea salt and cracked black pepper to season

Place the lime and lemon juice and chopped coriander in a large bowl and add the cod, monkfish and prawn. Mix together, cover and refrigerate for 30 minutes. Slowly melt the coconut oil and add the onion and garlic until transparent. Add the tomatoes, coconut milk, fish sauce, and cayenne pepper. Cover and simmer for 10 minutes. Then add the fish and juices and cook for 6-8 minutes. Garnish with lemon zest and chopped coriander.

Roasted Butternut Squash Soup

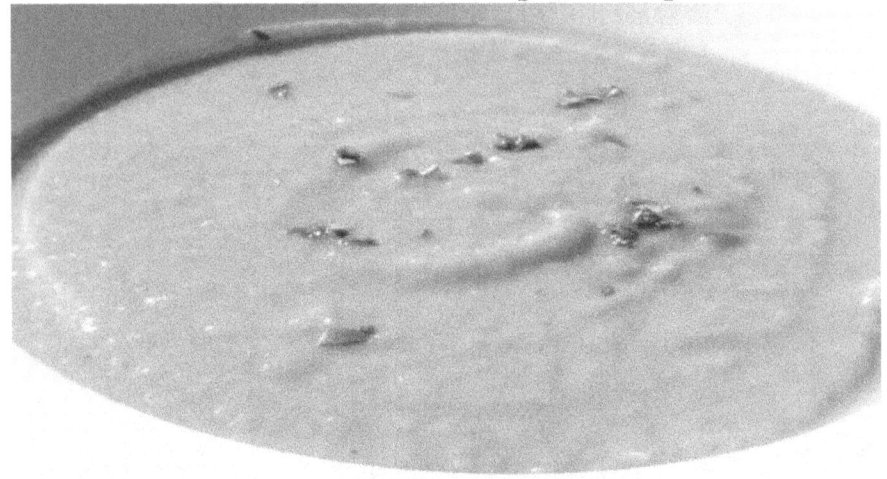

1 large butternut squash
1 green sliced apple
1 medium chopped onion
2 chopped carrots
3 tbsp olive oil
2 tsp cinnamon
½ tsp cumin
1 tsp chili powder
2 tbsp ghee or clarified butter
3 cups of vegetable or chicken stock

To prepare a butternut squash, first cut a thin slice off the bottom of the squash so that it can stand flatly. Then peel and using a sharp large knife, cut the squash in half lengthwise, and scoop out the seeds. Dice the peeled and seeded squash into cubes. In a large bowl combine the squash, olive oil, 1 tsp cinnamon, and ½ tsp cumin.

Mix together and spread out on a rimmed baking sheet. In the same bowl mix the apple slices, onion, and carrots and place on a second baking sheet. Put both sheets into a preheated oven and roast for 35-50 minutes until soft. Heat the butter gently in a large pot on the stove. Add the roasted ingredients and then the stock. Season with salt, pepper, cinnamon and a pinch of chili powder. Bring to a boil. Simmer for 20 minutes. Cool. Blend to a puree and re-heat and serve warm.

Sweet Potato and Bell Pepper Soup

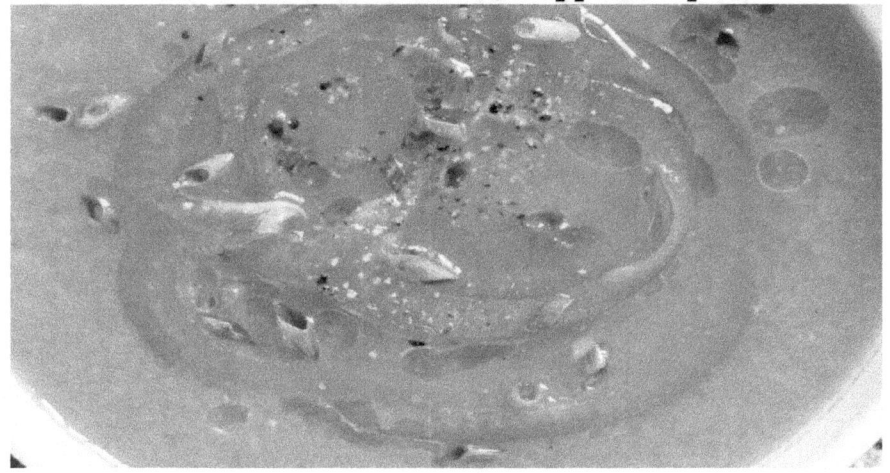

4 diced red bell peppers
4 cups of chicken stock
2 cups of mashed cooked sweet potato
1 diced onion
½ clove finely diced garlic
¼ teaspoon of finely diced ginger
1 tbl coconut oil
1 teaspoon ground cumin
juice of half a lemon
sea salt and cracked black pepper to season

Gently fry the onion, peppers and garlic in the coconut oil until transparent. Puree the mashed potato, ginger and stock and then add to the pan. Add the cumin, turn up the heat and simmer for 20 minutes. Add the lemon juice, and season to taste with salt and pepper. You can serve as is or blend it further to make it smoother.

Chicken Curry Soup

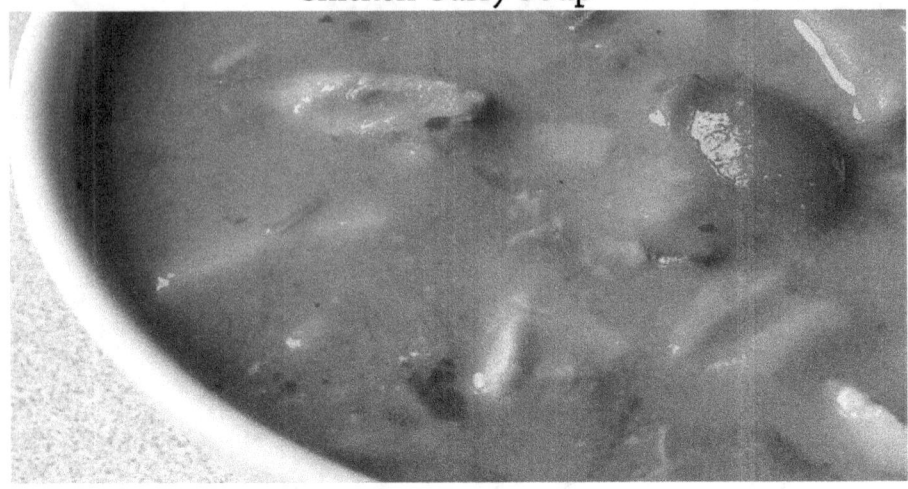

2 tablespoons coconut oil
½ sliced yellow onion
6 sliced green scallions
1 lb butternut squashed cubed
1 ln sweet potato cubed
1 red bell pepper
2 tablespoons of curry powder
2 tablespoons of tomato paste
1 tablespoon each of minced garlic, thyme and fresh ginger
1 can chopped tomatoes
4 cups of chicken or vegetable stock
2 teaspoons of Worcestershire sauce
1 can coconut milk
3 chicken breasts cut into thin strips
1/3 cup almond butter
2 tablespoons red wine vinegar
handful of chopped coriander and toasted almonds to garnish
sea salt and cracked black pepper to season

Gently fry the onion, scallions, pepper and garlic in the coconut oil until transparent. Add the sweet potato and squash and season. Cook until soft. Add the curry powder, tomato paste, ginger, and Worcestershire and combine well. Then throw in the stock, tomatoes and coconut. When it comes to the boil reduce hat and add the chicken, almond butter, and season. Cook for 20 minutes. Then finish with the red wine vinegar to taste. Garnish with chopped coriander and toasted almonds.

Tuscan Roasted Tomato Soup

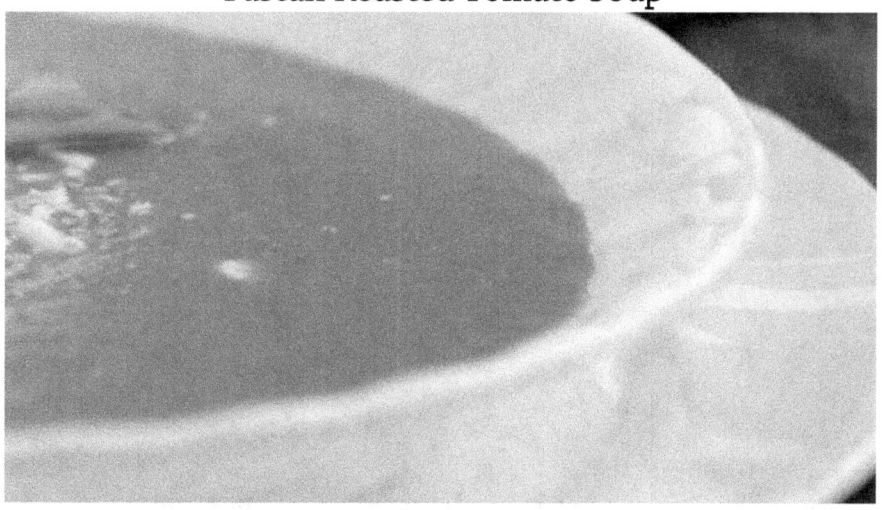

4 large vine tomatoes
1 medium onion
6 garlic cloves
1 tbsp olive oil
1 tbsp chopped flat leaf parsley
2 cups of vegetable or chicken stock
2 tbsp tomato paste
handful of chopped fresh basil leaves
sea Salt and cracked black pepper to season

Chop the tomatoes and onion into wedges, place in a bowl with the chopped garlic and basil, mix together with olive oil and then spread on a baking sheet.

Place in a pre-heated oven and bake for 30-40 minutes. Remove and cool. Heat the stock in a large pot, stir in the tomato paste and add the roasted tomatoes and simmer for 8-10. Allow cool and blend the puree until smooth. Season with salt and pepper.

Beef and Blueberry Stew

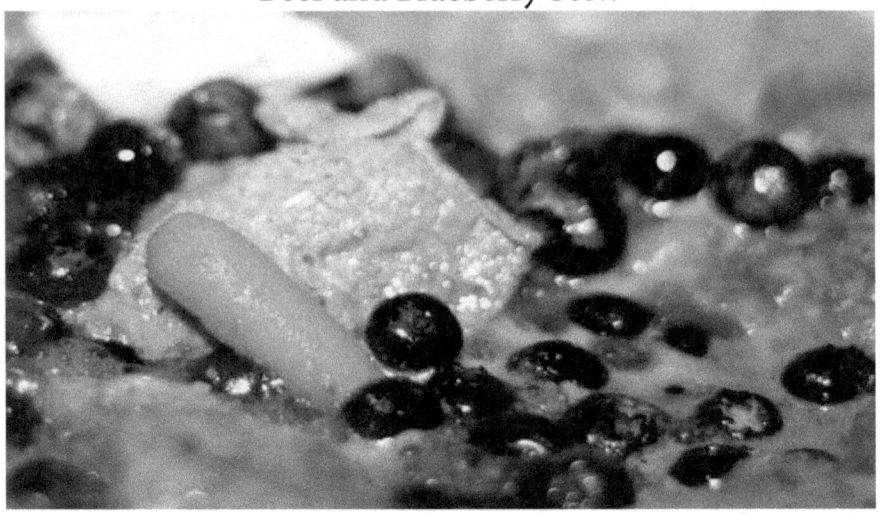

2 lb cubed sirloin beef
1 sliced onion
6 baby carrots
1 cup of fresh blueberries
1 clove garlic finely diced
Butter
coconut oil for frying
pinch of oregano
1 tablespoon of Worcestershire sauce
1 glass red wine

Fry the beef in coconut oil and then add the onions, carrots and garlic. Add the wine and Worcestershire sauce. Add water so that the meat is entirely covered. Stew for 30 minutes. Taste and season. Then add the berries and butter and mix through. Serve when the carrots and cooked.

Mango, Avocado and Chicken Salad

1 bag of shredded iceberg lettuce
2 boiled chicken breasts, shredded
1 peeled and diced mango
1 peeled, destoned and diced avocado
½ teaspoon of chili powder if you like it spicy
½ teaspoon cumin
juice of one lime
juice of ½ orange

2 tablespoons of olive oil
lime zest, sea salt and cracked black pepper to season

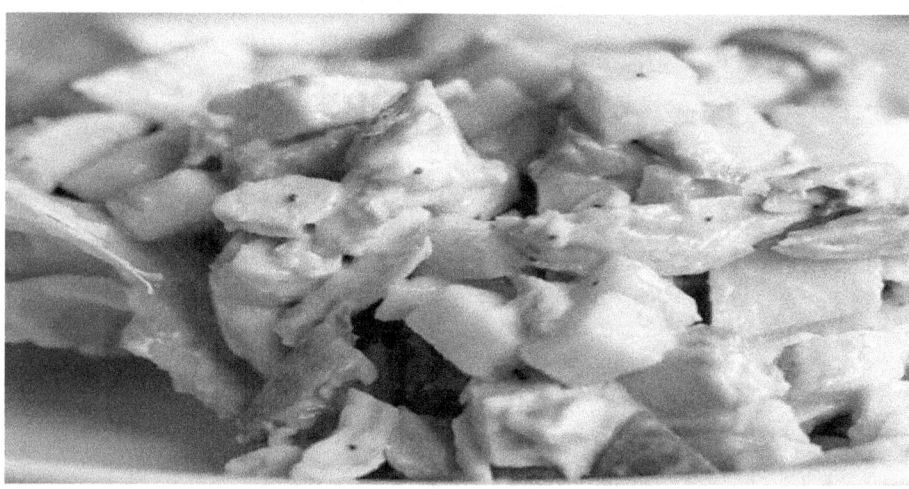

Place shredded chicken in a large bowl and mix with chili and cumin powder. Add the lime, orange, olive oil, diced mango and avocado and lettuce and gently mix all the ingredients together. Season with lime and orange zest.

Calamari Salad

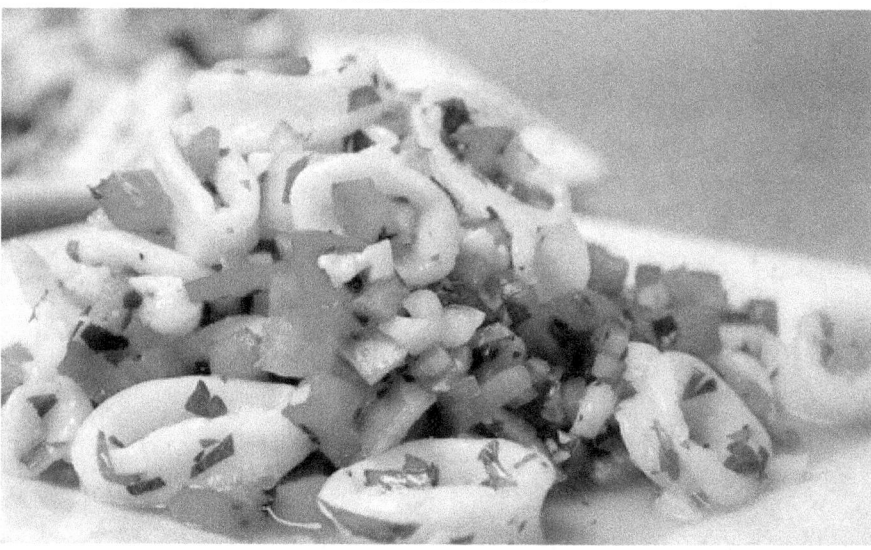

21/2 lbs frozen cleaned and trimmed raw calamari rings
3 tbls olive oil
3 minced garlic cloves
½ teaspoon of chili flakes
handful of chopped fresh mint leaves
handful of chopped coriander
handful of chopped flat leaf parsley
juice and zest of 1 lemon and one small orange
sea salt and cracked black pepper to season

Defrost calamari and rinse in cold water. Pat dry. Zest the fruit and cut six very thin slices from the rind. Heat the oil in a large pan (large enough to accommodate the calamari on one layer, if not, cook in batches). Add the calamari and garlic. Season. Cook for 4 minutes until opaque. Do not overcook! Drain and remove to a bowl. Add olive oil, chili, fruit juices, rinds and herbs and toss well. Season. Cover and chill until ready to serve. Sprinkle with the fruits zests.

Paleo Power Burger

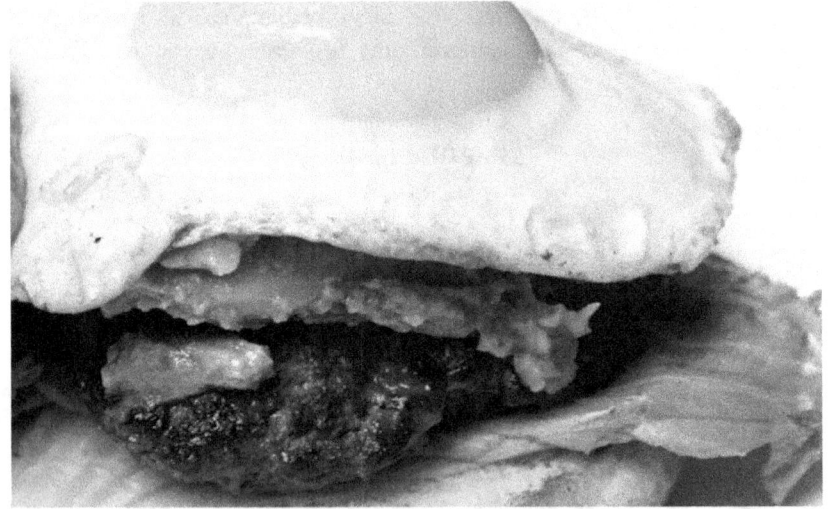

400 g grass fed or organic minced sirloin steak
50 g grass fed or organic minced pork
1 tbsp Dijon mustard
2 tbsp olive oil
4 cloves chopped garlic
1 chopped medium onion
1 beaten free range egg
1 chopped and de-seeded Jalapeno pepper

handful of chopped flat leaf parsley
2 tbsp chopped mint
1 teaspoon of finely chopped rosemary
2 slices of tomato
3 slices of avocado
1 free range egg of the mix
1 pan fried free range egg
sea salt and cracked black pepper

Fry the onion and garlic in olive oil and let them cool. In a large bowl mix together the mustard, Jalapeno pepper, egg, cooked garlic and onion, herbs, pork and beef. Season. Make into 3 or 4 patties and refrigerate for 30 mins. Then fry off and garnish with the tomatoes and avocado slices. Top with a fried egg.

Baked Peppers stuffed with Goat's Cheese or Brie

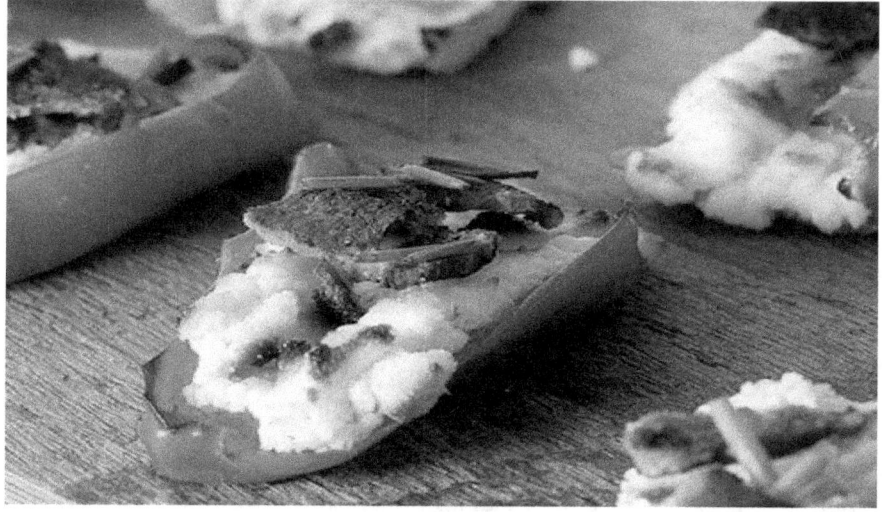

2 large red bell peppers cut into halves
8 oz goat's cheese or brie
½ cup ricotta cheese
8 sun dried tomatoes cut in half
1 finely chopped garlic clove
dash of tabasco
sea salt and cracked black pepper

Pre heat the oven and line a baking sheet with foil. Wash the peppers, discard seeds but leave the stem. Cut lengthways, cutting into the stems. In a bowl mix the Goat's cheese or Brie, the ricotta, tomatoes and the seasonings until well blended. Scoop the mixture into the peppers. Arrange the peppers on the baking sheet and roast for five minutes.

Beefburger stuffed with Avocado and sun dried Tomato

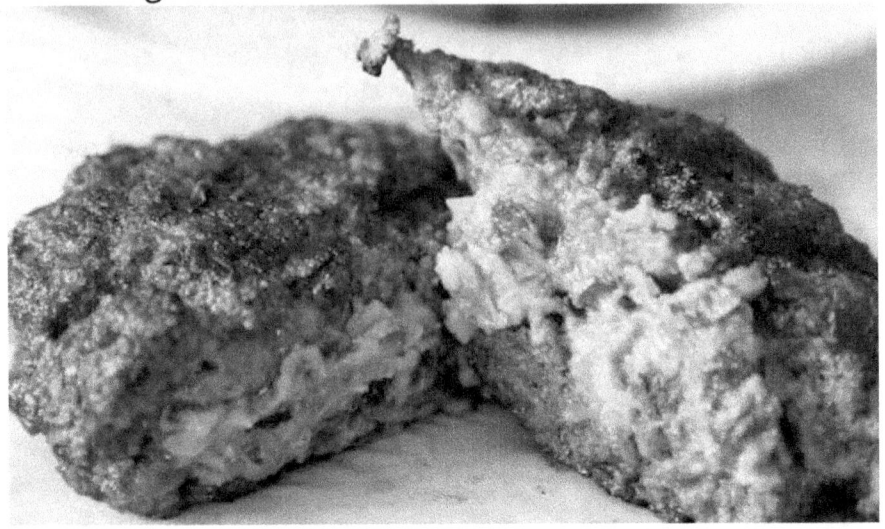

This recipe and photo are courtesy of cavemancooking.com
2 lbs organic minced beef
2 ripe avocados
1 cup of chopped sun-dried tomatoes, with NO OIL
juice of ½ lemon
zest of 1 lemon
1 tablespoon black pepper
2 teaspoons sea salt (makes it salty depending on your sun-dried tomatoes)

Preheat your grill to medium-medium high heat. Put your ground beef in a large mixing bowl and add black pepper, 1 teaspoon of sea salt, and the zest of one lemon. Mix well and then using your hands form into thin patties all the same size (you need them thin because you will be using two of them to make one patty). In another mixing bowl combine avocados, sun dried tomatoes, lemon juice, and the remaining teaspoon of sea salt. Mash the avocado and mix ingredients well to get as smooth as you like. Place your avocado mixture on top of the bottom of half of the burgers, ensuring you leave room to seal the burgers without it leaking out. Put your other patty over the top of your mixture and seal. Grill for about 6-8 minutes per side. Rest for ten minutes. You can use the rest of your avocado mixture to top your burgers.

Baked Salmon with Lemon

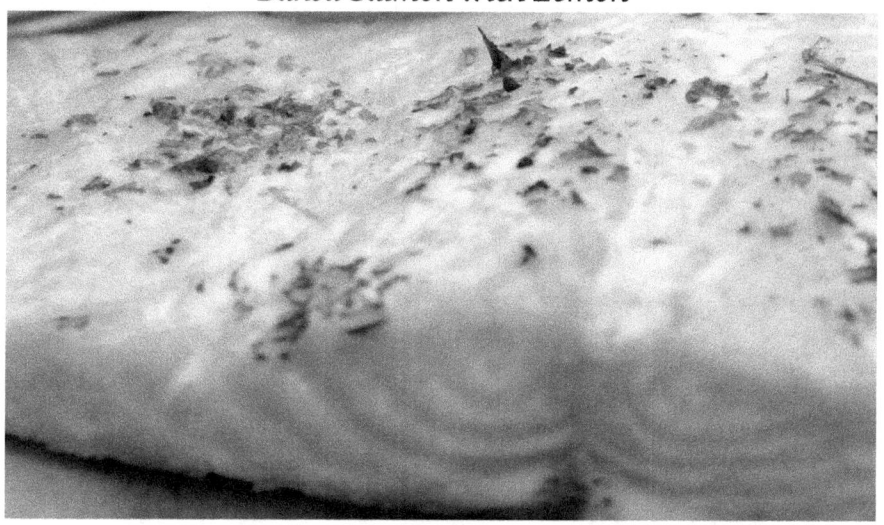

2 salmon darnes
1 lemon, sliced thin
1 tbsp capers
1 tbsp chopped fresh thyme
2 tbsp olive oil
sea salt and cracked black pepper

Line a baking sheet with parchment paper and place salmon, skin side down. Generously season salmon with salt and pepper. Arrange capers on the salmon, and top with sliced lemon and thyme. Place baking sheet in a cold oven, then turn heat to 400 degrees F. Bake for 25 minutes.

Mustard Pork Chops with Apricot and Apple Salsa

4 pork chops
½ cup of French mustard
6 apricots destoned
1 diced green apple
1 diced shallot
1 diced firm tomato
handful of shredded basil
3 tbsp raspberry vinegar
¼ cup of olive oil
1 tsp. ground cardamom
sea salt and cracked pepper to season

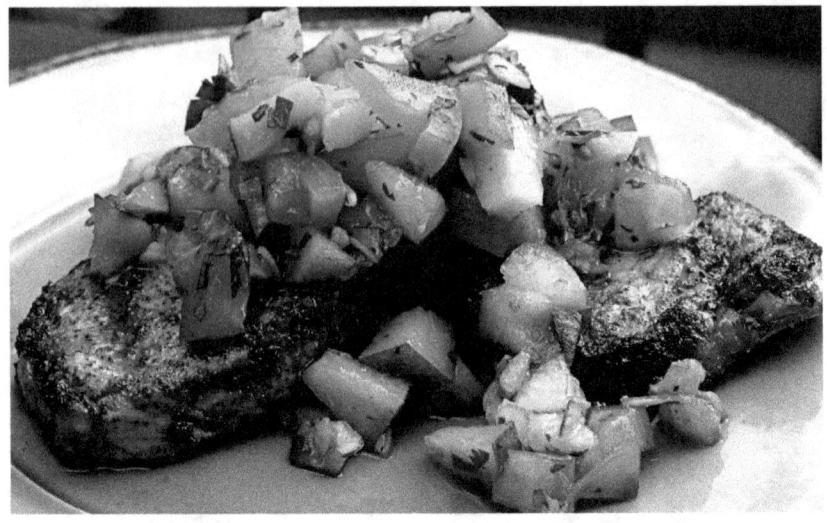

Season chops with salt and pepper on both sides and a little olive oil and cover with mustard. Mix all the other ingredients in a bowl. Grill the chops and continue to baste with mustard. When they are cooked serve with the salsa.

Shepherd's Pie

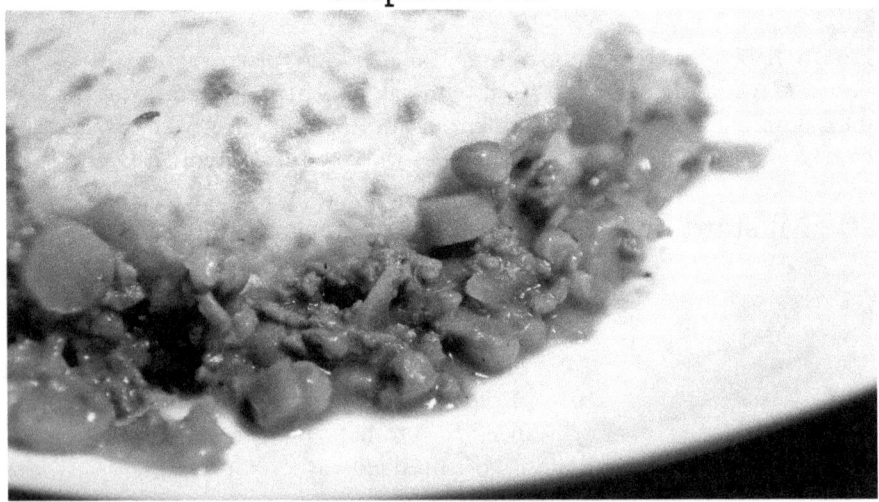

2 lbs minced organic lamb
4 cloves finely chopped garlic
1 diced onion

2 chopped carrots
12 sliced button mushrooms
1 cup of frozen peas
1 small can of tomato paste
2 tbsp balsamic vinegar
handful of chopped rosemary
handful of chopped thyme
4-6 baking or sweet potatoes
½ cup coconut milk
knob of butter
sea salt and cracked black pepper

Preheat your oven to 350 F. In a large skillet, brown the meat with the cloves of garlic in butter. Remove. Cook the onions, carrots and mushrooms until carrots are soft and onions are translucent. Return meat, add the tomato paste, balsamic vinegar, rosemary, and thyme. Season. Cook until the liquid evaporates. Stir in the peas. Pour the mixture into a large baking dish. Peel and boil the potatoes and then mash them with butter and the coconut milk. Spread on top of the meat mixture and bake for 20 minutes. Make sure the centre is piping hot. Shepherd's pie is always made with lamb – hence Shepherd!

Beef Kebabs

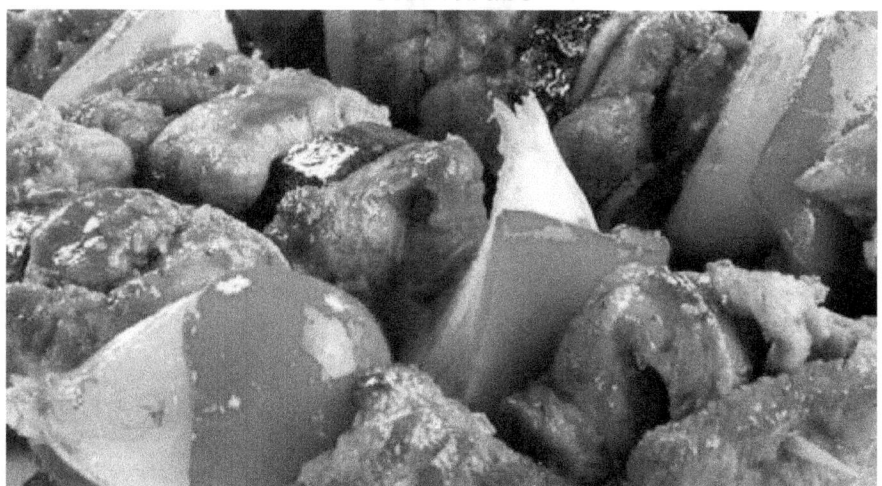

Marinade
1 chopped onion
5 chopped cloves of garlic
1 teaspoon orange zest
1 tbsp chopped rosemary

¼ cup fresh squeezed orange juice
¼ cup olive oil
2 tbsp organic tomato paste
Other Ingredients
2 lbs. sirloin, cut into 2 inch pieces
1 zucchini, cut into 1 inch rounds
1 yellow summer squash, cut into 1 inch rounds
1 red onion, cut into chunks
½ green bell pepper, cut into 1.5 inch chunks
½ red bell pepper, cut into 1.5 inch chunks

To make the marinade put all ingredients in a blender and blend until smooth. Reserve ¼ cup marinade for the vegetables. Place beef in a bowl and cover with the marinade. Toss to make sure it is well coated. Refrigerate for 4 hours to overnight. Remove the beef from the refrigerator 30 minutes before cooking, to allow it to come to room temperature. 30 minutes before grilling, toss the vegetables with the 1/4 cup reserved marinade. Remove the beef from the marinade and thread onto skewers. Do the same with the vegetables. Grill, turning every 5 minutes until the meat is pink and the vegetable cooked but firm.

THE MEDITERRANEAN DIET

WHAT IS IT?

The Mediterranean diet is based on the traditional foods that people used to eat in countries like Italy and Greece back in the 1960s. Studies showed that these people were exceptionally healthy compared to Americans and had a low risk of many killer diseases. We now know that this particular diet can cause weight loss and help prevent heart attacks, strokes, type II diabetes and premature death.

However, as there are many countries around the Mediterranean sea they don't all eat the same things. This article describes the diet that was typically prescribed in scientific studies that showed it to be an effective and healthy way of eating. There are several references to information received from the Mayo Clinic. If you're looking for a heart-healthy eating plan, this diet may be the right one for you as it includes the basics of healthy eating and allows you drink red wine, a real plus if you're a wino like me.

As you know, the majority of healthy diets include fruits, vegetables, fish and whole grains, and limit unhealthy fats. While these parts of a healthy diet are well tested, subtle variations in proportions of certain foods may make a difference in your risk of heart disease. Many studies have proven that the traditional Mediterranean diet reduces the risk of heart disease.

In fact, an analysis of more than 1.5 million healthy adults demonstrated that following a Mediterranean diet was associated with a reduced risk of death from heart disease and cancer, as well as a reduced incidence of Parkinson's and Alzheimer's diseases. As well as that, the Dietary Guidelines for Americans fully endorses this diet as an eating plan.

THE KEY COMPONENTS
The Mediterranean diet emphasizes:
- Eating primarily plant-based foods, such as fruits and vegetables, whole grains, legumes and nuts. Residents of Greece average six or more servings a day of antioxidant-rich fruits and vegetables. Nuts are another part of a healthy Mediterranean diet. Nuts are high in fat, but most of the fat is healthy. Because nuts are high in calories, they should not be eaten in large amounts, generally no more than a handful a day. For the best nutrition, avoid candied or honey-roasted and heavily salted nuts.
- Replacing butter with healthy fats, such as olive oil. Throughout the Mediterranean region, bread is eaten plain or dipped in olive oil not eaten with butter or margarine, which contains saturated or trans fats.
- Using herbs and spices instead of salt to flavor foods.
- Limiting red meat to no more than a few times a month.
- Eating fish and poultry at least twice a week.
- Daily exercise.
- Drinking red wine in moderation (optional)

WHAT ARE THE BASIC FOODS YOU CAN EAT?
EAT PLENTY OF: All kinds of Vegetables, Fruits, Nuts, Legumes, Potatoes, Whole Grains, Herbs, Spices, Fish particularly shellfish and Olive Oil.
VEGETABLES
Tomatoes, broccoli, kale, spinach, onions, cauliflower, carrots, Brussels sprouts, and cucumbers.
FRUITS
Apples, bananas, oranges, pears, strawberries, grapes, dates, figs, melons, and peaches.
LEGUMES
Beans, peas, lentils, pulses, peanuts, and chickpeas.
TUBERS
Potatoes, sweet potatoes, turnips, and yams.
WHOLE GRAINS
Whole oats, brown rice, rye, barley, corn, buckwheat, whole wheat, whole grain bread and pasta.
NUTS AND SEEDS
Almonds, walnuts, Macadamia nuts, hazelnuts, cashews, sunflower seeds, pumpkin seeds and more. Nuts and seeds are good sources of fiber, protein and healthy fats. Keep almonds, cashews, pistachios and walnuts on hand for a quick snack. Choose natural peanut butter, rather than the kind

with hydrogenated fat added. Try blended sesame seeds (tahini) as a dip or spread for bread.

SEAFOOD

Salmon, sardines, trout, tuna, mackerel, shrimp, oysters, clams, crab, and mussels. Fatty fish like mackerel, lake trout, herring, sardines, albacore tuna and salmon are rich sources of omega-3 fatty acids. Fish is eaten on a regular basis in the Mediterranean diet. Eat fish at least twice a week. Grill, bake or broil fish for great taste and easy cleanup. Avoid breaded and fried fish.

HEALTHY OILS

Olive oil, avocado oil, olives and avocadoes. The diet features olive oil as the primary source of fat. Olive oil is mainly monounsaturated fat which is a type of fat that can help reduce low-density lipoprotein (LDL) cholesterol levels when used in place of saturated or trans fats. "Extra-virgin" and "virgin" olive oils (the least processed forms) also contain the highest levels of protective plant compounds that provide antioxidant effects.

Canola oil and some nuts contain the beneficial linolenic acid (a type of omega-3 fatty acid) in addition to healthy unsaturated fat. Omega-3 fatty acids lower triglycerides, decrease blood clotting, and are associated with decreased incidence of sudden heart attacks, improve the health of your blood vessels, and help moderate blood pressure.

EAT A LITTLE OF:

Poultry, eggs, cheese and yogurt. Choose low-fat dairy. Limit higher fat dairy products, such as whole or 2 percent milk, cheese and ice cream. Switch to skim milk, fat-free yogurt and low-fat cheese.

EAT VERY LITTLE OF:

RED MEAT

Cut down on red meat. Limit red meat to no more than a few times a month. Substitute fish and poultry for red meat. When choosing red meat, make sure it's lean and keep portions small (about the size of a deck of cards). Also avoid sausage, bacon and other high-fat, processed meats.

DO NOT EAT

Sugar-sweetened beverages, added sugars, processed meat, refined grains, refined oils and other highly processed foods. In particular, we're talking about the following:

SUGARS

Sodas, candies, ice cream and table sugar.

REFINED GRAINS

Including white bread and pasta made with refined wheat.

TRANS-FATS
Trans fats in margarine and various processed foods.
REFINED OIL
Like soybean oil, canola oil, and cottonseed oil.
PROCESSED MEATS
All processed meat particularly sausages, frankfurters, and hot dogs..
LABELS
Watch out for anything labelled "low-fat" or "diet" or looks like it was made in a factory.

WHAT TO DRINK
Water should be your go-to beverage on a Mediterranean diet. This diet also includes moderate amounts of red wine, that is, limited to one glass per day. Coffee and tea are also completely acceptable, but avoid sugar-sweetened beverages and fruit juices, which are very high in sugar.

SIMPLE MEAL PLANNERS BUT ALSO CHECK THE RECIPES
As with the paleo diet I am going to give you set daily meal plans for six mini meals. Again, the planner is a template, so switch it around to suit yourself. And don't forget to try some of the delicious recipes.

	SUNDAY
BREAKFAST	Scrambled Eggs on Rustic Bread
ELEVEN	Greek Yogurt and Strawberries
LUNCH	Pasta Salad
AFTERNOON	Cup of mixed Nuts and Raisins
DINNER	Prawn and Pasta
NIGHT-TIME	Cup of chopped Almonds and Raisins
TREATS	Either glass of Wine or two squares of Chocolate (70%)

	MONDAY
BREAKFAST	Vegetable Omelette (Peppers, Onions, Tomatoes etc) cooked in olive oil
ELEVEN	Cup of mixed Nuts and Raisins
LUNCH	Tomato, Red Onion, Olives and Feta Salad
AFTERNOON	Slice of Cheese and sliced Pear
DINNER	Grilled Salmon
NIGHT-TIME	Banana
TREATS	Either glass of Wine or two squares of Chocolate (70%)

	TUESDAY
BREAKFAST	Greek Yogurt with sliced Strawberries
ELEVEN	Diced Avocado and Tomato
LUNCH	Sardines with Tomato and Cucumber Salsa
AFTERNOON	Cup of mixed Nuts and Raisins
DINNER	Mediterranean Pizza
NIGHT-TIME	Cup of Cherries
TREATS	Either glass of Wine or two squares of Chocolate (70%)

	WEDNESDAY
BREAKFAST	Two Fried Eggs and Red Peppers cooked in olive oil
ELEVEN	Greek Yogurt and Berries
LUNCH	Mediterranean Panini made with Italian Rustic Bread
AFTERNOON	Slice of Cheese and sliced Pear
DINNER	Stuffed Tomatoes See Recipe
NIGHT-TIME	Turkey Slices
TREATS	Either glass of Wine or two squares of Chocolate (70%)
	THURSDAY
BREAKFAST	Whole Grain Sandwich with Cheese
ELEVEN	Avocado and Tomato Salsa
LUNCH	Tuna Salad
AFTERNOON	Greek Yogurt and chopped Apple
DINNER	Artichokes alla Romana
NIGHT-TIME	Banana
TREATS	Either glass of Wine or two squares of Chocolate (70%)

	FRIDAY
BREAKFAST	Greek Yogurt and Banana
ELEVEN	Cup of mixed Nuts and Raisins
LUNCH	Stuffed Tomatoes
AFTERNOON	Cup of Cherries
DINNER	Stuffed Portobello Mushrooms
NIGHT-TIME	Turkey Slices
TREATS	Either glass of Wine or two squares of Chocolate (70%)

	SATURDAY
BREAKFAST	Vegetable Omelette (Peppers, Onions, Tomatoes etc) cooked in olive oil
ELEVEN	Greek Yogurt and chopped Apple
LUNCH	Stuffed Roasted Peppers
AFTERNOON	Slice of Cheese and sliced Pear
DINNER	Tuna Salad
NIGHT-TIME	Banana
TREATS	Either glass of Wine or two squares of Chocolate (70%)

15 DELICIOUS MEDITERRANEAN RECIPES

Scrumptious Panini

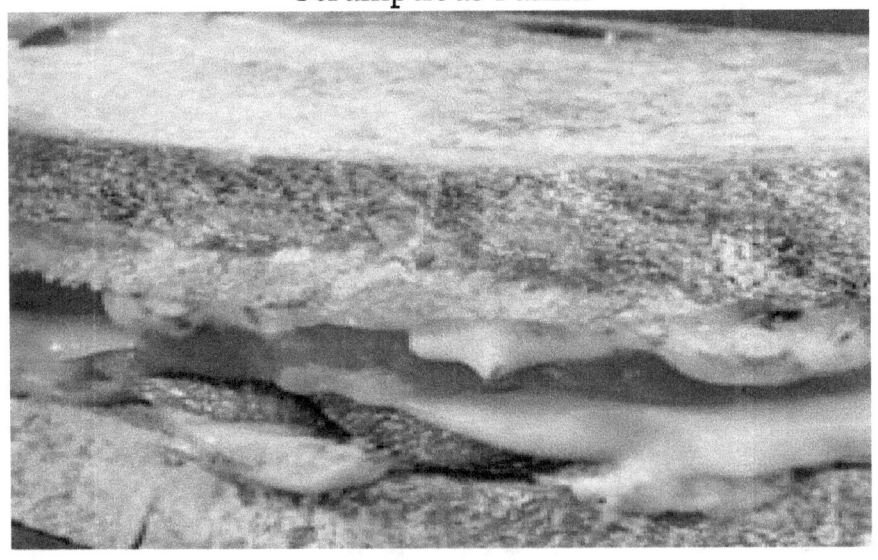

½ cup of Greek yogurt
handful of chopped fresh basil leaves
2 tablespoons finely chopped oil-cured black olives
8 slices rustic whole grain bread (about 1/2-inch thick)
1 thinly sliced courgette
4 slices provolone cheese
1 sliced roasted roasted red pepper
4 grilled streaky rashers

Mix the yogurt, basil with olives in small bowl. Evenly spread bread slices with yoghurt, then layer 4 bread slices with courgette, provolone, peppers and rashers. Top with remaining 4 bread slices. Spread remaining yogurt on the outside of sandwiches and grill for five minutes until sandwiches are golden brown and cheese is melted.

Greek Tuna Salad

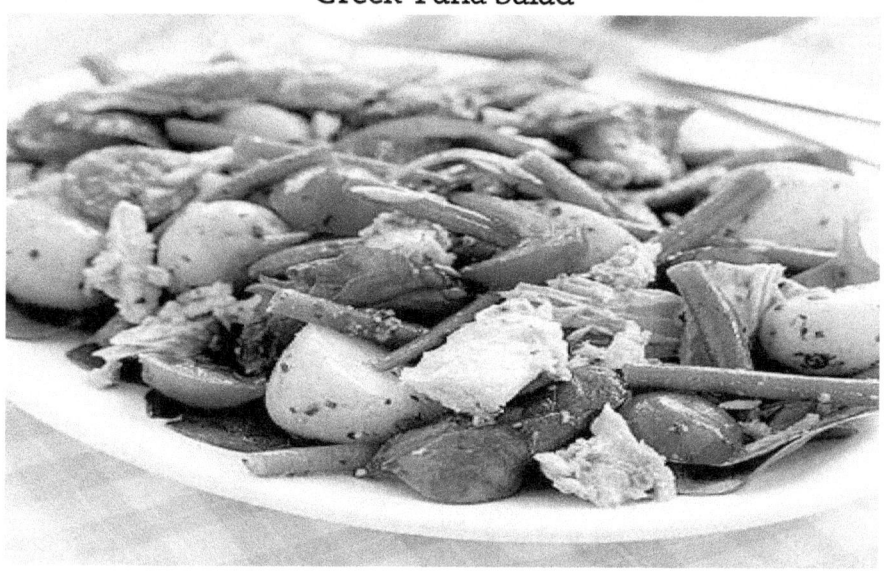

1 pound boiled but firm French green beans cut into thirds
1 medium sized can of tuna packed in oil
¼ cup extra-virgin olive oil
8 cherry tomatoes quartered
juice of ½ lemon
1 teaspoon anchovy paste
2 tablespoons black olives
handful of torn fresh flat-leaf parsley leaves
8 boiled baby potatoes cut in half
sea salt and cracked black pepper to season

Wait until the beans and potatoes have cooled down to a warm temperature. Then gently mix all the ingredients in a bowl and serve. You can top this dish with a fried egg for color and presentation.

The Best Vegetarian Lasagne Ever
Courtesy of the Guardian newspaper. www.guardian.co.uk.

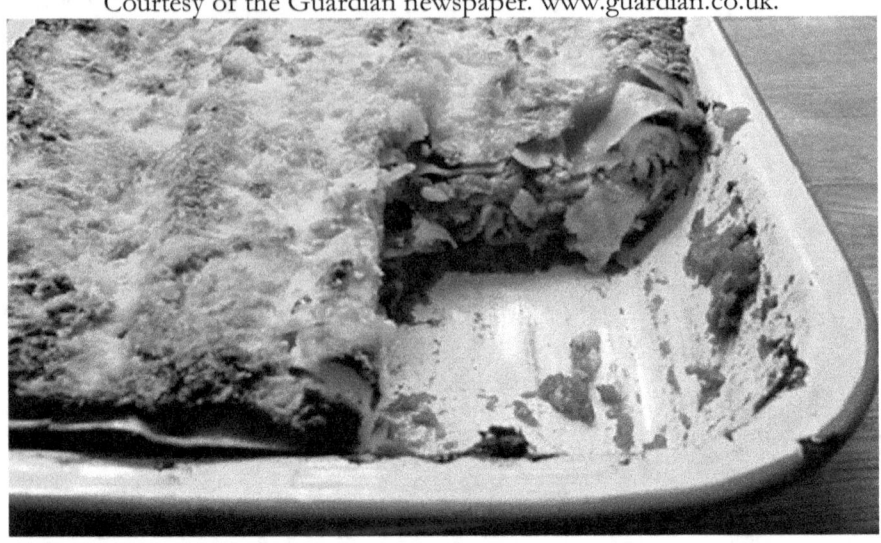

This recipe serves six
3 aubergines
2 red peppers
50g pine nuts
2 tbsp olive oil
2 garlic cloves, crushed
600g chopped tomatoes
Slug of balsamic vinegar
500g ricotta
75g pecorino Romana (or parmesan), finely grated
12 dried lasagne sheets or 6 fresh ones
small bunch of basil, leaves picked

Heat the oven to 200C/400F/gas mark six. Prick the aubergines and put the aubergines and peppers on a lightly greased baking tray and bake for about 40 minutes until charred and collapsing in on themselves. Put the pine nuts in the oven for the last five minutes to toast.

When the aubergines and peppers are cool enough to handle, scoop out the flesh of the aubergines and mash up any large pieces. Peel the peppers, remove the seeds and finely chop the flesh, then add to the aubergine. Heat the oil in a frying pan and sauté the garlic for a minute or so. Add the aubergine and pepper mixture and fry for about 10 more minutes, stirring fairly frequently, until you have a thick pulp, then add the tomatoes and a generous slug of balsamic vinegar. Rinse out the tomato tins with a little water and add this to the pan as well. Bring to the boil, then simmer for about 10 minutes until reduced. Season to taste. Mix the ricotta with the toasted pine nuts and about three-quarters of the pecorino. Season to taste. If you're using dried pasta, blanch in boiling salted water for about a minute until just floppy. To assemble the lasagne, spread a quarter of the aubergine mixture in the base of a shallow oven dish (about 20cm x 25cm) and top with a few torn basil leaves and a layer of pasta, cutting it to fit if necessary. Spread with just under a quarter of the ricotta mixture and add another quarter of the aubergines, and some more basil. Repeat these layers (ricotta, aubergine, basil, pasta) twice more, finishing off with a thicker layer of ricotta. Sprinkle with the remaining cheese and bake for about 35-40 minutes until golden brown.

Baked Salmon with Salsa

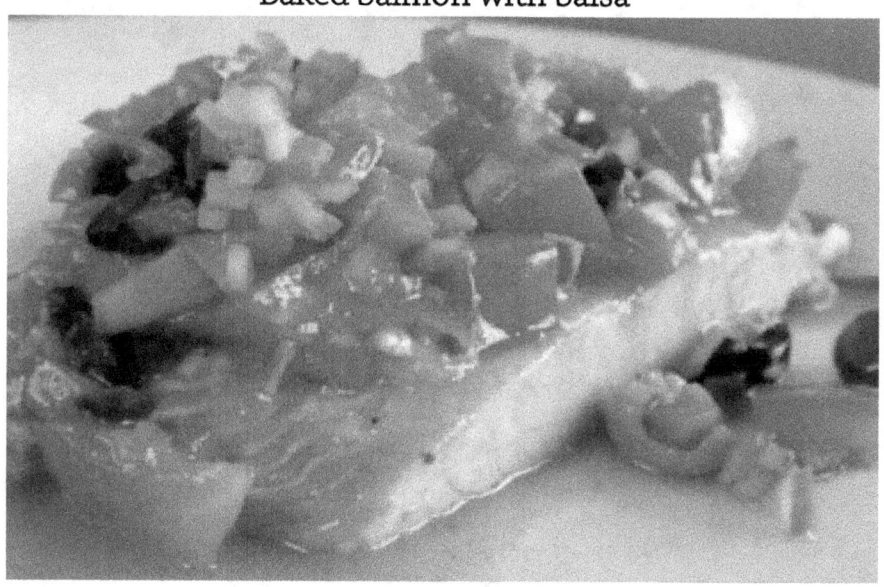

4 salmon fillets
¼ cup sliced pitted black olives
¼ cup chopped red bell pepper
¼ cup chopped red onion
8 cherry tomatoes, quartered
1/4 cup sun-dried tomato vinaigrette dressing

Preheat oven to 400°F. Place salmon, skin side down, on foil-lined baking sheet and gently coat with olive oil. Bake for 18-20 minutes. Mix remaining ingredients in a bowl and spoon over salmon.

Stuffed Portobello Mushroom

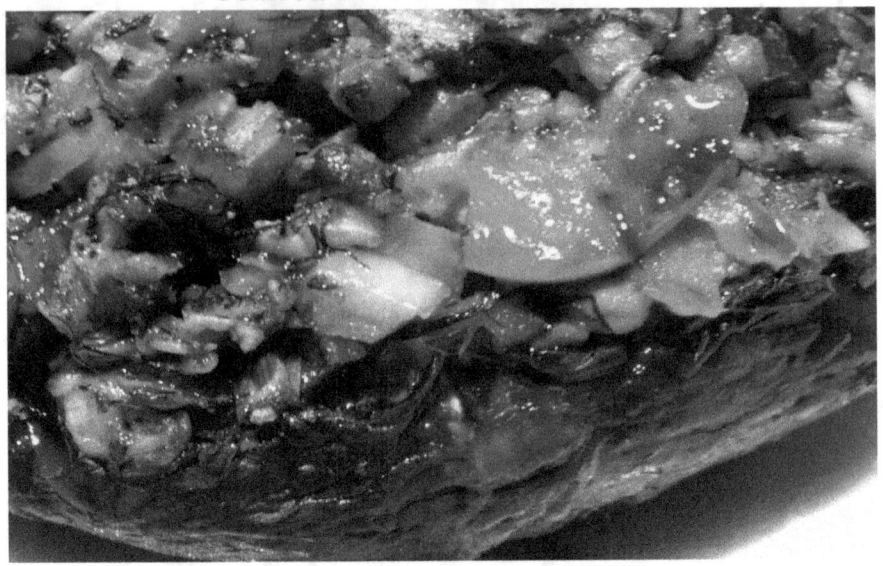

Marinated mushrooms
1 cup olive oil
½ cup balsamic vinegar
½ soy sauce
2 minced garlic cloves
4 large fresh thyme sprigs
6 large portobello mushrooms
sea salt and cracked black pepper to season
Filling
1 packet of spinach
1 pound button mushrooms
2 tablespoons olive oil
1 cup chopped onion
3 minced garlic cloves
6 tablespoons finely grated Parmesan cheese
¼ cup unseasoned dry breadcrumbs
½ slice of feta cheese crumbled

For marinated mushrooms: Cut stems from mushrooms and place stems in a processor with thyme and a little stock. Arrange mushrooms, gill side up, and pour marinade over mushrooms and marinate 4 hours, turning to coat occasionally.

For filling: Cook spinach in a little olive oil and set aside. Add half of button mushrooms to processor with portobello mushroom stems. Transfer to medium bowl and repeat with remaining mushrooms. Heat oil and sauté onion and garlic. Then add chopped mushrooms. Cook. Season and transfer to large bowl. Cool.. Then add spinach, a little Parmesan, and breadcrumbs to mushroom mixture. Add feta cheese and season. Cover filling and let stand at room temperature. Preheat oven to 400°F. Transfer marinated mushrooms on a baking tray gill side down. Roast until beginning to soften, about 15 minutes. Turn mushrooms over. Divide filling among mushrooms. Sprinkle remaining 6 tablespoons Parmesan cheese over and bake until heated through and cheese begins to brown.

Farfalle Pasta Salad

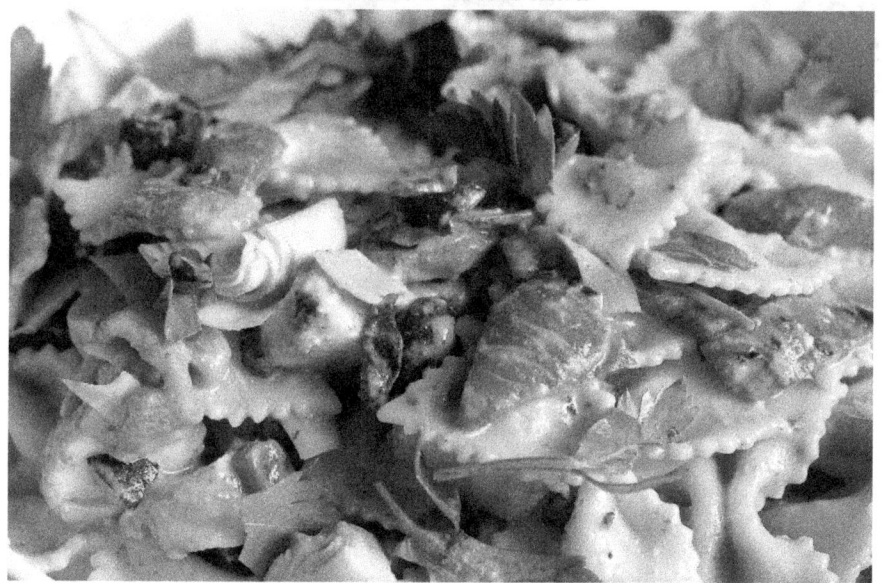

1 yellow and 1 red bell pepper de-seeded and diced.
1 diced onion
1 cup frozen peas, thawed and cooked in boiling water for 3 minutes
3 thinly sliced scallions
½ cup pf black olives
1 tablespoon olive oil
1 pound farfalle pasta
1 cup prepared pesto
¼ cup freshly grated Parmesan cheese
sea salt and cracked black pepper

Mix the peppers, onion, peas, scallions, and olives in a bowl. Reserve. Cook the pasta and drain. Reserve ¼ cup of pasta water. Add the pesto and reserved vegetables to the pasta. Toss with cheese and season.

Eat Yourself Thin Detox Salad

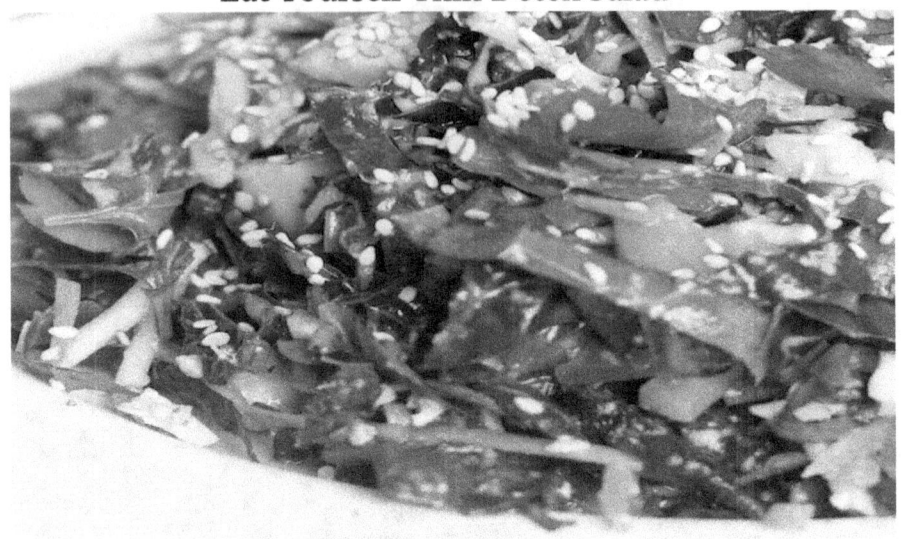

Salad
2 cups of shredded red cabbage
2 cups of shredded kale
½ cup of chopped flat leaf parsley
1 roasted red pepper diced
2 cups of chopped broccoli
1 carrot cut into matchsticks
1 cut of chopped walnuts
2 sliced avocados
2 teaspoons sesame seeds
Sea salt and cracked black pepper to season
Dressing
juice of ½ lemon
juice of ½ orange
½ cup of olive oil
1 teaspoon of minced ginger
1 teaspoon of agave nectar
Shot of tabasco

In a bowl mix the dressing ingredients. In another bowl mix the salad ingredients. Toss dressing with vegetables until well mixed. Transfer to a serving bowl and top with sesame seeds and season.

Crab Salad

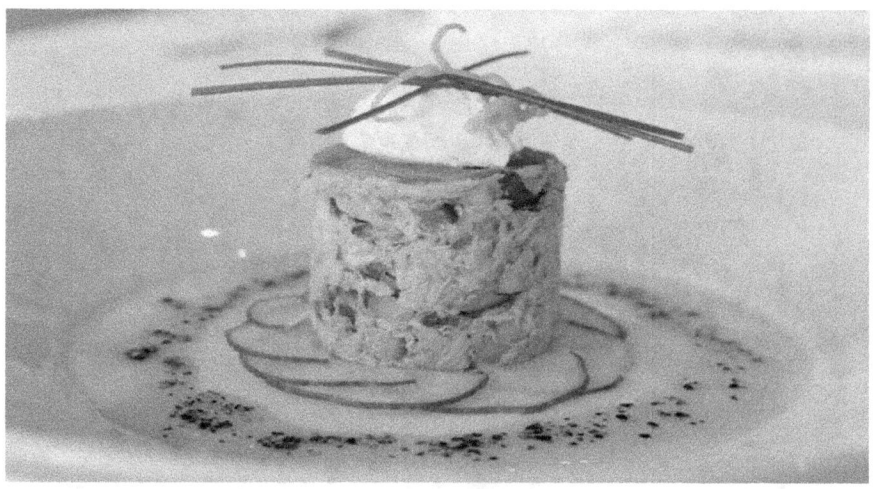

1 packet of crab meat
½ cup of Greek yoghurt or no fat mayo
juice of ¼ lemon
teaspoon of French mustard
dash of tabasco
½ finely chopped skinned green apple
½ stalk of celery finely chopped
2 inches of cucumber finely chopped
smoked salmon
chives
crème fraiche
sea salt and cracked black pepper

This looks a lot more complicated than it actually is. Mix all the ingredient together and season with sea salt and cracked black pepper. Place in a metal ring and refrigerate for 30 minutes. Drain and serve. Top with sliced of smoked salmon, chives and a dollop of crème fraiche on a bed of thinly sliced cucumber.

Three Bean Salad

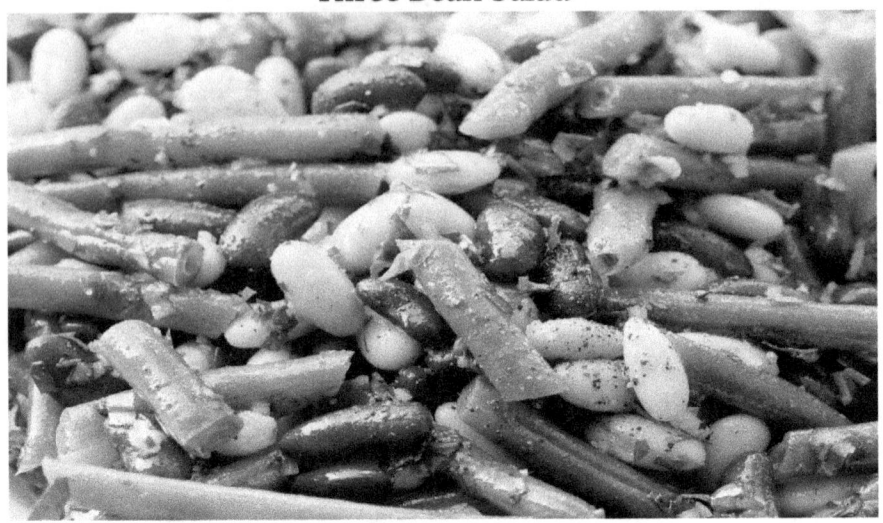

1 X 15oz can of chickpeas
1 X 15oz can of kidney beans
Large handful of French beans – boil and keep, then chop in 1 inch sizes
handful of chopped flat leaf parsley
2 chopped scallions
1 chopped red onion
1 chopped celery stick
½ cup olive oil
½ cup wine vinegar
1 tablespoon of soy
1 tablespoon honey
½ teaspoon of dried mustard
½ clove minced garlic
dash of tabasco
juice of ½ lemon
sea salt and cracked black pepper to season

Mix all the ingredients together.

Lime Steamed Kale

12 cups of chopped Kale
Dressing
juice of 1 lime
3 minced garlic cloves
1 tablespoon extra virgin olive oil

1 teaspoon soy
sea salt and cracked pepper

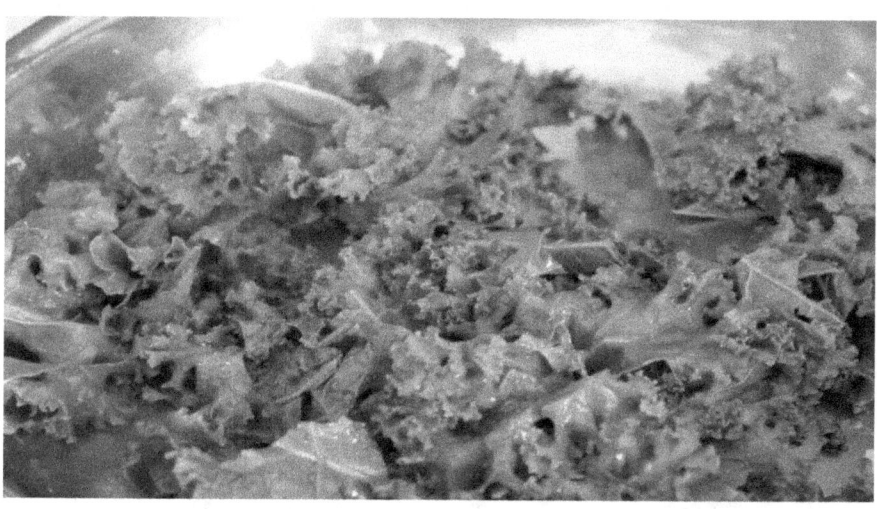

Wash and steam the Kale for 7-10 minutes. In a bowl whisk all the ingredients together and then add the Kale. Toss and serve warm.

Greek Roasted Peppers

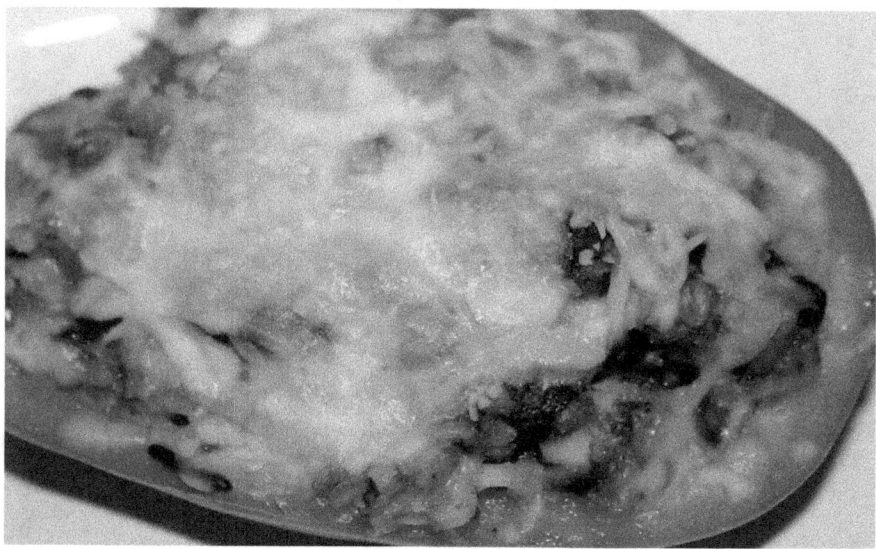

1 pound lean ground beef
handful of spinach leaves
1 thinly diced courgette
1 diced shallot
1 egg, lightly beaten
$\frac{1}{2}$ teaspoon dried oregano
sea salt and cracked black pepper
3 red pepper cut in half
1 can chopped tomatoes
$\frac{1}{2}$ cup of chopped feta and red cheddar cheese

Preheat the oven to 350 degrees F. Mix the beef, spinach, courgette, shallot, egg, oregano, salt and a few grinds of pepper. Mix until thoroughly combined. Place the peppers on a baking dish and fill with the mixture. Pour the tomatoes over the peppers and sprinkle with the cheese. Cover with foil and bake for 30 minutes. Uncover and bake for 30 minutes until the meat mixture is completely cooked and the peppers are tender.

Mussels and Potatoes

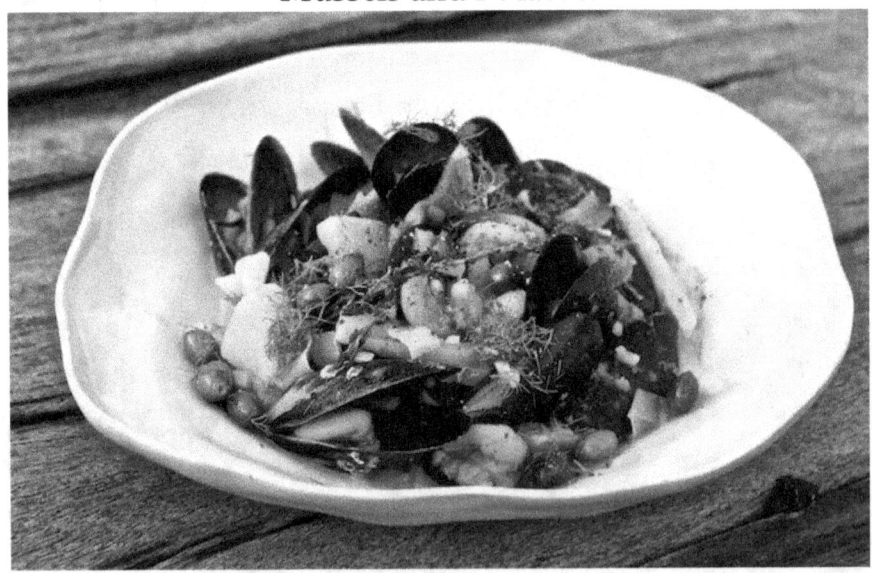

2 large potatoes cut into cubes
2 tablespoons olive oil
1 medium sliced onion
4 cloves chopped garlic
$\frac{1}{2}$ teaspoon paprika

pinch of cayenne pepper
1 can diced tomatoes
2 1/4 pounds mussels, scrubbed
2/3 cup halved pitted green olives
handful of chopped flat leaf parsley
glass of white wine

Boil the potatoes and then chop. Heat the olive oil and add the onion and garlic and cook until soft and golden brown. Add the potatoes, paprika, cayenne and season. Stir in the wine and the tomatoes. Bring to a simmer, cover and cook until the potatoes are tender, about 10 minutes. Stir in the mussels, olives and parsley. Cover and cook until the mussels open, 4 to 5 minutes. Discard any mussels that do not open.

Baked Stuffed Tomatoes

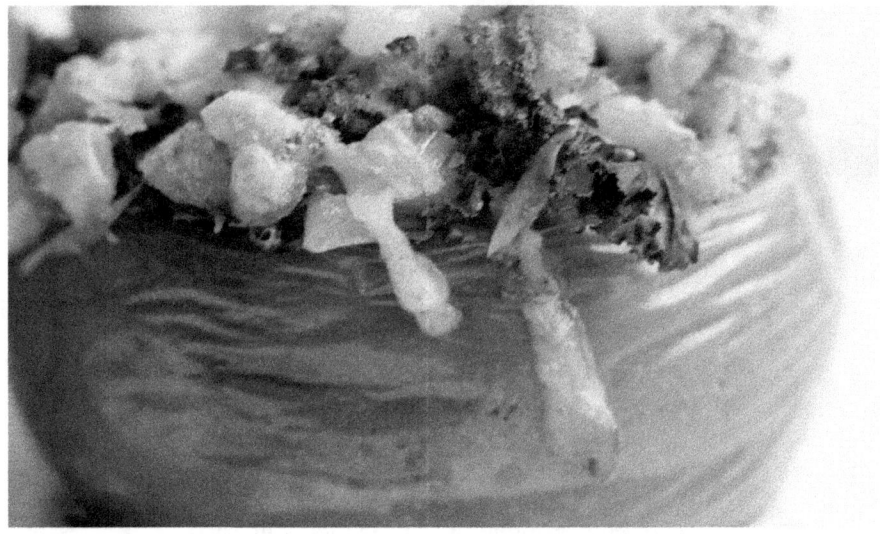

2 large plum tomatoes
½ cup garlic croutons
¼ cup of crumbled feta cheese
¼ cup of sliced pitted kalamata olives
2 tablespoons olive oil
1 tablespoon of balsamic vinegar
2 tablespoons chopped fresh basil
sea salt and cracked black pepper

Preheat the oven. Cut tomatoes in half crosswise. Use your finger to push out the pulp and discard the seeds. Chop the pulp and place in a bowl.

Place hollowed tomatoes, cut sides down, on a paper towel and drain for a few minutes. Add croutons, feta cheese, olives, dressing, and basil to pulp; mix well. Season with sea salt and cracked black pepper. Mound mixture into hollowed tomatoes. Place tomatoes on a baking sheet and bake for 5 minutes until hot, the cheese melts and the croutons are crispy.

Spaghetti with Prawn and crumbled Feta Cheese

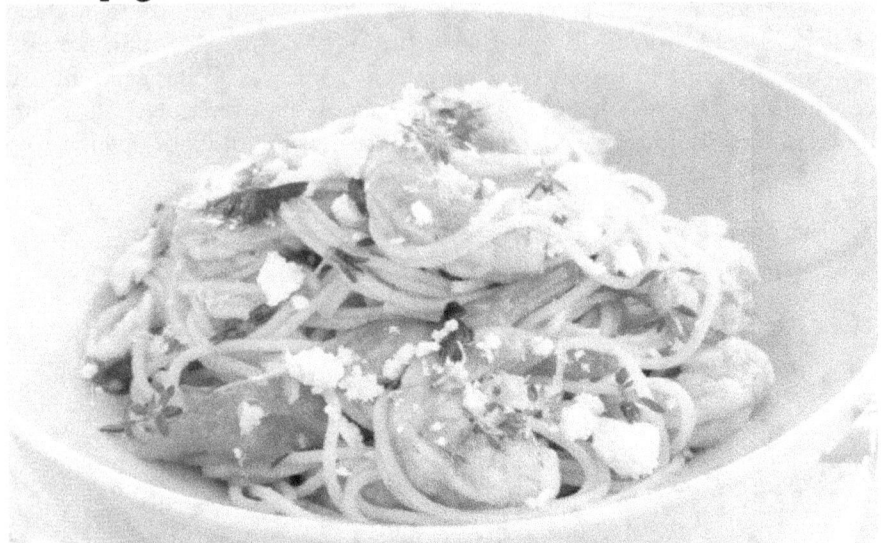

¼ cup of olive oil
3 finely diced garlic cloves
1 pound medium prawn/shrimp, peeled and deveined
2 cups chopped plum tomato
handful of finely torn fresh basil
handful of torn flat leaf parsley
¼ cup chopped pitted kalamata olives
1 tablespoon drained capers
4 cups hot cooked whole wheat (preferably) spaghetti
2 ounces crumbled feta cheese (optional)
sea salt and cracked black pepper

Heat olive oil in a large pan and sauté the garlic for 30 seconds. Add prawn/shrimp and sauté 1 minute. Add tomato and basil; reduce heat, and simmer for 3 minutes or until tomato is tender. Stir in kalamata olives, capers, salt and black pepper. Combine prawn/shrimp mixture and pasta in a large bowl; toss well. Top with cheese and sprigs of parsley and serve.

Mediterranean Chicken Wrap

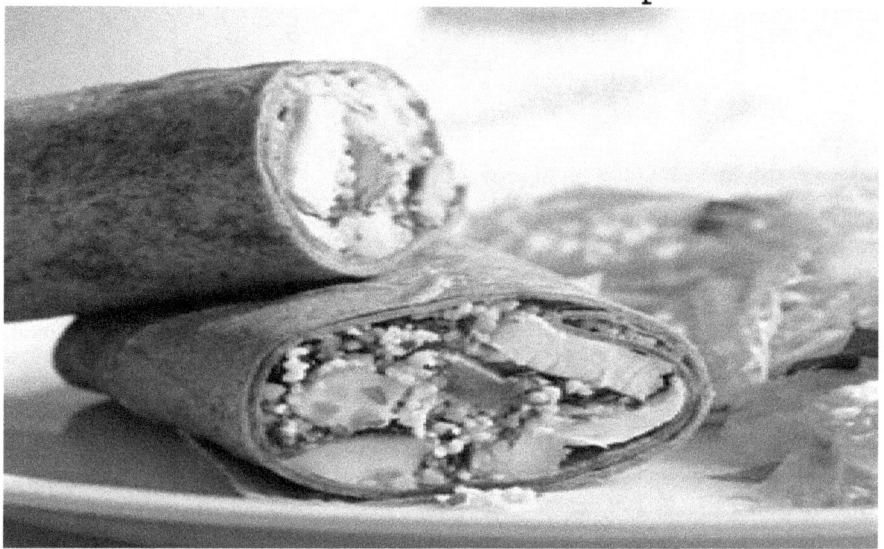

This recipe is courtesy of www.eatingwell.com.

2 cups water
½ cup whole wheat couscous
handful of torn flat leaf parsley
handful of torn mint
juice of half lemon
¼ cup olive oil
2 cloves finely chopped garlic
2 chicken breasts, boiled and cut into bite size pieces
1 chopped tomato
1 cup chopped cucumber
4 X 10-inch spinach wraps or tortillas
sea salt and cracked black pepper to season

Bring water to a boil in a saucepan. Stir in couscous and remove from heat. Cover and let stand for 5 minutes. Fluff with a fork and set aside. Mix the parsley, mint, lemon juice, oil, garlic in a bowl and season. Mix the couscous with tomato and cucumber. Divide the mixtures and chicken between the wraps. Roll them up, tucking in the sides. Cut in half and serve.

THE LOW CARB DIET

WHAT IS IT?

A low carb involves eating natural, unprocessed foods with a low carbohydrate content and emphasizes foods high in protein and fat. Scientific studies prove that this type of diet is one of the best options for people who want to lose weight, optimize health and lower the risk of disease. However, what foods you should eat depends on how healthy you are, how much exercise you take and how much weight you have to lose.

There are many types of low-carb diets. Some of these diets may have health benefits beyond weight loss, such as reducing risk factors associated with diabetes and metabolic syndrome. People choose the low-carb diet if they want a diet that restricts certain carbs to help lose weight or if they want to change their overall eating habits or simply enjoy the type of foods featured in low-carb diets.

As the name suggests, a low-carb diet restricts the carbohydrates you eat. What are carbohydrates? Carbohydrates are a type of calorie-providing macronutrient found in many foods and beverages. Many carbohydrates occur naturally in plant-based foods like grains. In natural form, carbohydrates can be thought of as complex and fibrous such as the carbohydrates found in whole grains and legumes, or they can be less complex such as those found in milk and fruit. The common sources of naturally occurring carbohydrates include grains, milk, nuts, fruits, vegetables, seeds and legumes like beans, peas and lentils.

Food manufacturers also add refined carbohydrates to processed foods in the form of flour or sugar. These are generally called simple carbohydrates.

Examples of these include white breads, pasta, biscuits and cookies, cake and candy, and sugar-sweetened sodas and drinks. Our bodies use carbohydrates as their main source of fuel. Sugars and starches are broken down into simple sugars during digestion. They're then absorbed into our bloodstream, where they are known as blood sugar (glucose). Fiber-containing carbohydrates resist digestion. Despite the fact they have less effect on blood sugar, complex carbohydrates provide bulk and serve other body functions beyond fuel.

When blood sugar levels rise it causes the body to release insulin. Insulin helps glucose enter our body's cells. Some glucose is used by our body for energy and fuels all of our activities, whether it's walking or simply breathing. Extra glucose is usually stored in our liver, muscles and other cells for later use or it is converted to fat. The reason why people use low-carb diet is because by decreasing carbs you lower insulin levels. This causes the body to burn stored fat for energy and ultimately leads to weight loss.

Generally speaking, a low-carb diet will focus on proteins like meat, poultry, fish and eggs, and some non starchy vegetables. Again, generally, it will exclude or limit most grains, pastas and starchy vegetables, fruits, legumes, breads, sweets, and sometimes nuts and seeds. Some low-carb diet plans allow small amounts of certain fruits and vegetables. A daily limit of 60 to 130 grams of carbohydrates is the norm of a low-carb diet. These amounts of carbohydrates provide 240 to 520 calories.

A very low-carb diet will restrict carbohydrates to 60 grams or less a day. In contrast, the Dietary Guidelines for Americans recommend that carbohydrates make up 45 to 65 percent of your total daily calorie intake. Accordingly, you should note that if you consume 2,000 calories a day, you would need to eat between 900 and 1,300 calories a day from carbohydrates or between 225 and 325 grams of carbohydrates per day. A word of warning first.

If you suddenly and drastically cut your carbohydrate intake, you may experience a variety of side effects like bad breath, fatigue, headaches, constipation or diarrhea. In fact, some diets restrict carbohydrate intake so much that in the long term they can result in vitamin or mineral deficiencies, bone loss, and gastrointestinal disturbances and may increase risks for various chronic diseases. If you were to restrict your carbohydrate intake to less than 20 grams a day you be be warned that this can result in a process called ketosis.

Ketosis occurs when you don't have enough sugar (glucose) for energy, so your body breaks down stored fat, causing ketones to build up in your body. Side effects from ketosis include bad breath, general nausea, headaches, as well as mental and physical fatigue. Exactly what kind of possible long-term health risks a low-carb diet may pose is uncertain. This is because most research studies have lasted less than a year.

Some studies suggest that if you eat large amounts of fat and protein from animal sources your risk of heart disease or certain cancers may actually increase. But there are definite benefits. Most people lose weight in the short term on diet plans that restrict calories and what you can eat. And very low-carb diets may lead to greater short-term weight loss than low-fat diets. But most studies have found that at twelve or twenty four months, the benefits of a low-carb diet are not great. Basically, it's a short term weight loss strategy.

WHAT YOU SHOULD EAT
MEAT
Beef, lamb, pork, chicken and others. Grass-fed is best.
FISH
Salmon, trout, haddock and many others. Wild-caught fish is best.
EGGS
Omega-3 enriched or pastured eggs are best.
VEGETABLES
Spinach, broccoli, cauliflower, carrots and many others.
FRUIT
Apples, oranges, pears, blueberries, strawberries.
NUTS AND SEEDS
Almonds, walnuts, and sunflower seeds.
HIGH FAT DAIRY
Cheese, butter, heavy cream, yogurt.
FATS AND HEALTHY OILS
Coconut oil, butter, lard, olive oil and cod fish liver oil.

WHAT YOU SHOULD NOT EAT
SUGAR
Soft drinks, fruit juices, agave, candy, ice cream and many others.
ARTIFICIAL SWEETENERS
Aspartame, Saccharin, Sucralose, Cyclamates and Acesulfame Potassium. Use Stevia instead.
GLUTEN GRAINS
Wheat, spelt, barley and rye. Includes breads and pastas.
SEED OILS
Cottonseed oil, soybean oil, sunflower oil, grapeseed oil, corn oil, safflower

oil and canola oils.
TRANS FATS
"Hydrogenated" or "partially hydrogenated" oils.
LABELS
Be careful of anything labelled "diet" and low-fat products and highly processed foods. Many dairy products, cereals, crackers, etc

WHAT TO DRINK
Water, Coffee, Tea and Carbonated soda without artificial sweeteners.

SIMPLE MEAL PLANNERS BUT ALSO CHECK THE RECIPES
As with the previous two diets I am going to give you set daily meal plans for six mini meals. Again, the planner is a template, switch it around to suit yourself. And don't forget to try some of the delicious recipes.

	SUNDAY
BREAKFAST	Greek Salad Omelette fried in Butter
ELEVEN	Organic Yogurt with Berries
LUNCH	Spicy Chicken Wings with Yogurt Dip or Salsa (see recipe)
AFTERNOON	Low Carb Smoothie (Coconut Milk, Berries, Almonds and Protein powder)
DINNER	Prawn and Avocado Cocktail
NIGHT-TIME	Banana
TREATS	Either glass of Wine or two squares of Chocolate (70%)

	MONDAY
BREAKFAST	Bacon and Eggs fried in Butter
ELEVEN	Smoothie
LUNCH	BEATS Salad
AFTERNOON	Apple
DINNER	Garlic Spinach
NIGHT-TIME	Full Fat Yogurt
TREATS	Either glass of Wine or two squares of Chocolate (70%)

	TUESDAY
BREAKFAST	Eggs and Red Pepper fried in Butter
ELEVEN	Organic Yogurt and Strawberries
LUNCH	Oriental Lettuce wrap (see recipe)
AFTERNOON	Smoothie
DINNER	Chicken Marengo
NIGHT-TIME	Banana
TREATS	Either glass of Wine or two squares of Chocolate (70%)

	WEDNESDAY
BREAKFAST	Tomato and Cheese Omelette fried in Butter
ELEVEN	Smoothie
LUNCH	Prawn, Bacon and Avocado Salad (see recipe)
AFTERNOON	Apple
DINNER	Garlic Lemon Broccoli
NIGHT-TIME	Turkey slices
TREATS	Either glass of Wine or two squares of Chocolate (70%)

	THURSDAY
BREAKFAST	Eggs and Red Peppers fried in Butter
ELEVEN	Organic Yogurt and Berries
LUNCH	Ranch Chicken BLT Salad (see recipe)
AFTERNOON	Smoothie
DINNER	Prawn Bacon and Avocado Salad
NIGHT-TIME	Banana
TREATS	Either glass of Wine or two squares of Chocolate (70%)

	FRIDAY
BREAKFAST	Greek Salad Omelette fried in Butter
ELEVEN	Smoothie
LUNCH	Chicken Wings with Yogurt dip or Salsa
AFTERNOON	Apple
DINNER	BEATS Salad
NIGHT-TIME	Turkey slices
TREATS	Either glass of Wine or two squares of Chocolate (70%)

	SATURDAY
BREAKFAST	Bacon and Eggs fried in Butter
ELEVEN	Banana
LUNCH	BEATS Salad
AFTERNOON	Smoothie
DINNER	Ranch Chicken BLT Salad
NIGHT-TIME	Full Fat Yogurt
TREATS	Either glass of Wine or two squares of Chocolate (70%)

15 LOW CARB DIET RECIPES

BEATS Salad

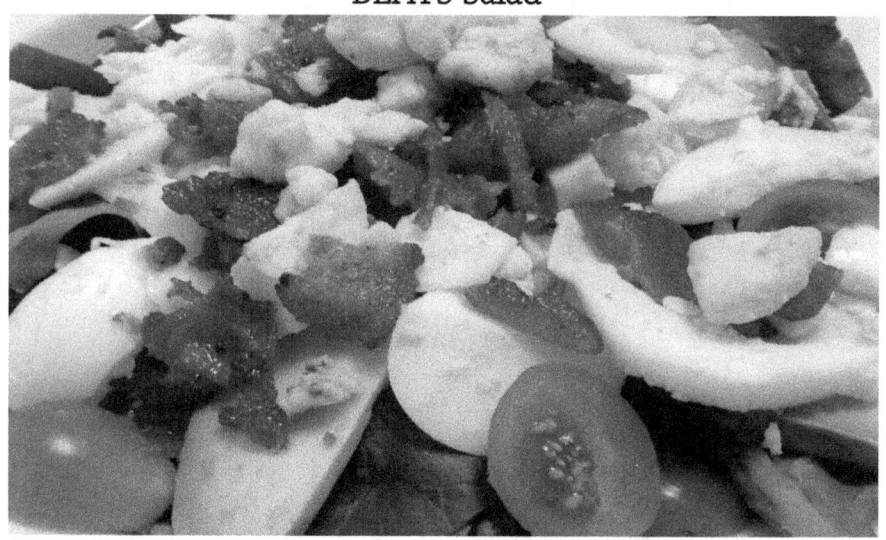

4 slices of fried bacon chopped into small pieces
2 diced boiled eggs
1 ripe diced avocado
1 medium-sized diced tomato
juice of ¼ lime
sea salt and cracked black pepper to season

Gently mix all the ingredients together and serve.

Oriental Lettuce Wrap

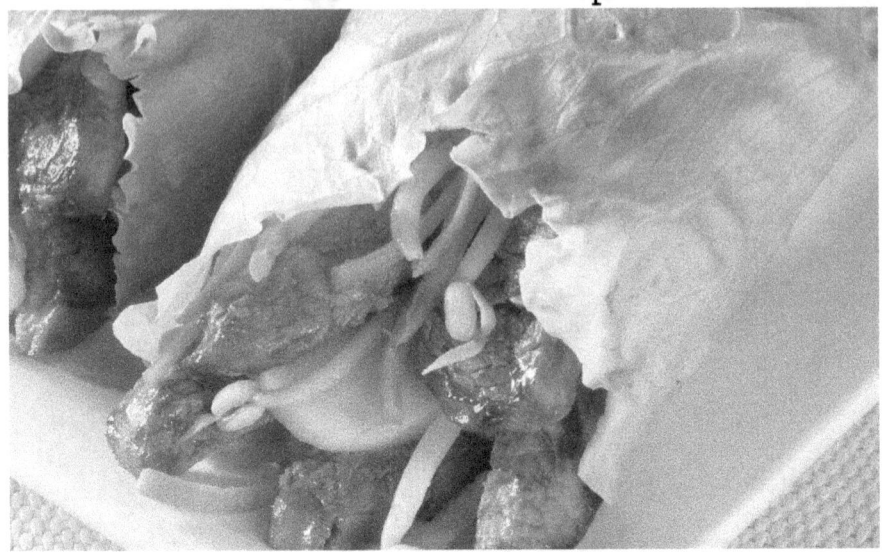

1 pound of pork loin cut into slices
4 oz mushrooms
½ diced onion
3 finely chopped cloves garlic
2 chopped scallions
handful of bean sprouts
handful of coriander
½ cup of carrots very thinly sliced into matchsticks
juice of 1 lemon
1 teaspoon of chili garlic sauce
1 tablespoon of soy
1 tablespoon of sesame oil
iceberg lettuce

Sauté the pork in oil. In a bowl add the lemon juice, chili sauce, soy, scallions, beansprouts and coriander and mix. Let the pork cool a little and add to the mixture. In the frying pan add a little oil and cook the mushrooms, onion and garlic Then add to the mixture. Divide the mixture between cups of your lettuce and wrap.

Ranch Chicken BLT Salad

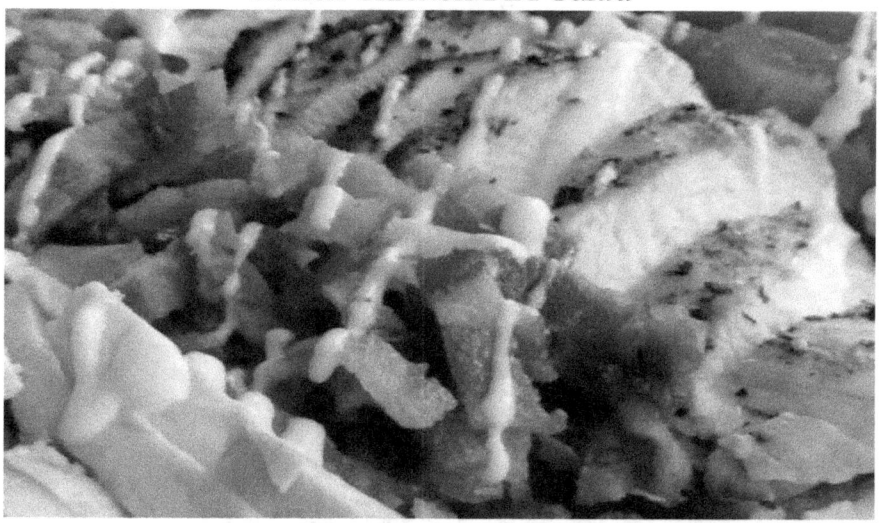

1 grilled boneless chicken breast, grilled
2 cups of torn iceberg lettuce
1 small chopped tomato
½ oz Swiss cheese cut into thin slices
2 slices of streaky bacon cut into pieces
1 hard boiled sliced egg
sea salt and cracked black pepper to season
Ranch Dressing
1 cup mayonnaise
½ cup sour cream
½ teaspoon dried chives
½ teaspoon dried parsley
½ teaspoon dried dill weed
¼ finely diced garlic clove
½ finely diced shallot
sea salt and cracked black pepper to season

Whisk all the ingredient together to make this delicious sauce.

Either place all the salad ingredients side by side on a plate as in the picture or mix together. Drizzle the Ranch sauce over it.

Spicy Chicken Wings

This is a very simple dish. Take a dozen chicken wings. Cover with Hot Sauce and lime juice. Bake in the oven and serve with a tomato, cucumber and avocado salsa. Alternatively serve with a Full Fat Yoghurt dip.

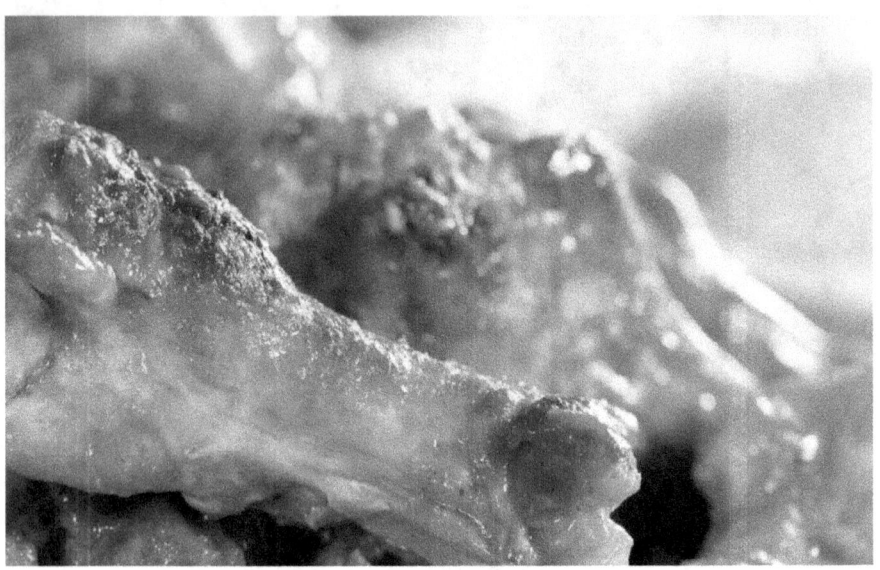

Bacon Prawn and Avocado Salad

Dressing
juice of one half lime
2 tablespoons of extra virgin olive oil
½ cup of torn coriander
sea salt and cracked black pepper to season
Mix all ingredients in a bowl..
Salad
1 pound of cooked prawns/shrimp
2 ripe sliced avocados
2 slices of streaky bacon sliced
½ cup of garlic croutons
4 cups green lettuce
(You can add some red lettuce for color if you like)

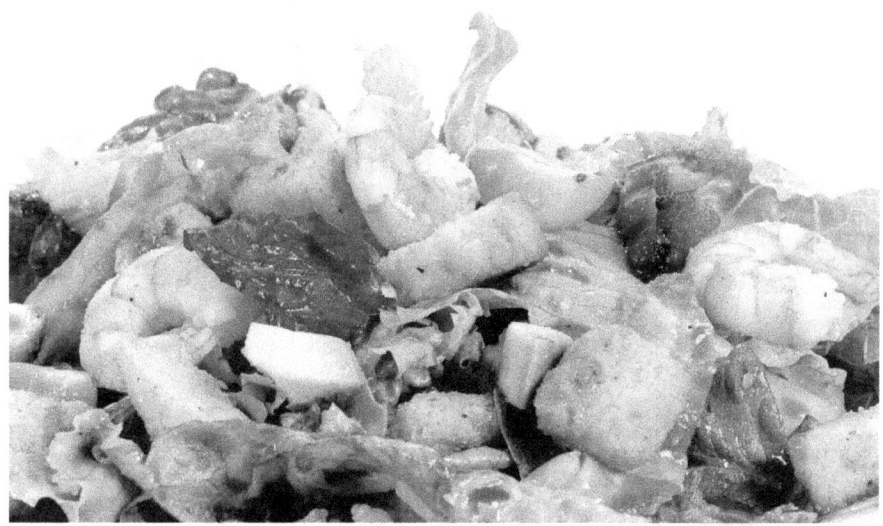

Marinate the prawns in the dressing and refrigerate for one hour. Make up the salad and then pour the prawns and marinade over the salad and mix.

Garlic Spinach

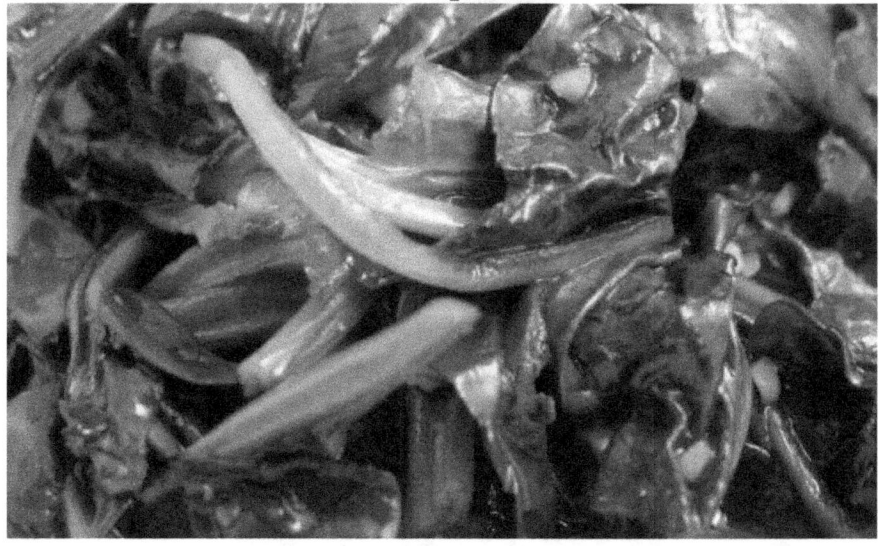

1 bag of washed fresh spinach
2 cloves of finely chopped garlic
½ cup of extra virgin olive oil
1 large tomato finely diced

1 teaspoon of finely diced ginger
juice of ½ lime
2 tablespoons of balsamic vinegar

This is quite a substantial dish so you easily have it for your dinner at night. I like it with balsamic tomato but that's optional. Put the tomato into a bowl and cover with the balsamic. Put the spinach in a hot wok and season with the oil, garlic, ginger, salt and pepper. Stir it until it begins to wilt and then add the lime juice. Just before serving mix though the tomato.

Garlic Lemon Broccoli

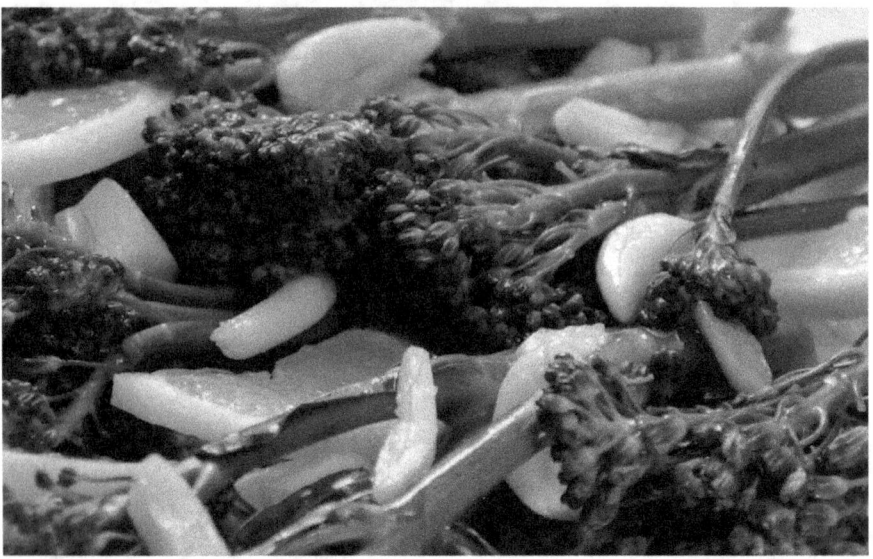

1 head of broccoli cut into bitesize florets
4 cloves of split garlic
½ cup of extra virgin olive oil
juice of ½ lemon and the juice of ¼ orange
½ lemon cuts into slices
½ teaspoon of grated nutmeg
sea salt and cracked black pepper

Put the broccoli into a pan and add boiling water. Boil for 3 minutes. Drain and cover with iced water. Pat it dry with kitchen paper. Put some oil in the pan and add the sliced garlic. Cook for a few minutes and then add the broccoli. Pour over the oil and mix until each part of the broccoli is covered with oil. Turn up the heat and add the fruit juices. Take off the pan, plate and grate nutmeg over it. Serve with lemon slices.

Greek Salad Omelette

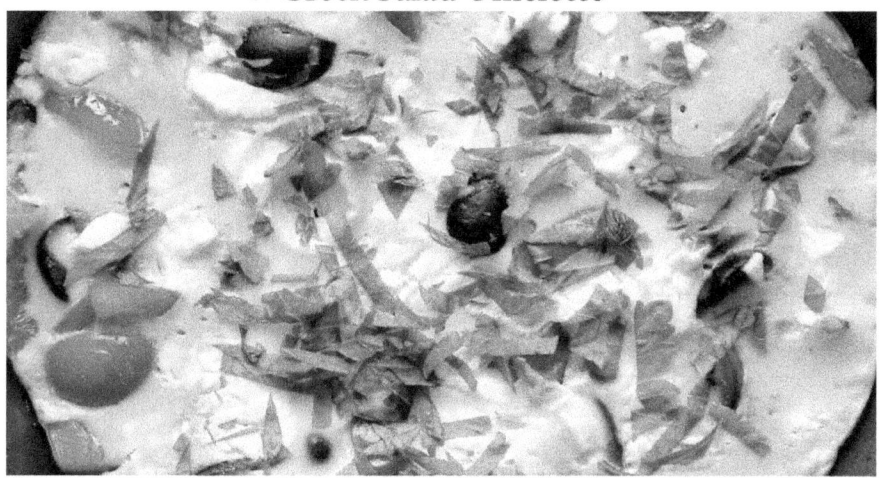

5 free range or omega 3 eggs
handful of chopped flat leaf parsley
2 tbsp olive oil
1 medium red onion, cut in strips wedges
2 vine tomatoes
½ cup of pitted black olives cut in half
50g feta cheese, crumbled
sea salt and cracked black pepper to season

Heat the grill to high. Whisk the eggs in a large bowl with the chopped parsley, pepper and salt, if you want. Heat the oil in a large non-stick frying pan, then fry the onion wedges over a high heat for about 4 mins until they start to brown around the edges.

Throw in the tomatoes and olives and cook for 1-2 mins until the tomatoes begin to soften. Turn the heat down to medium and pour in the eggs. Cook the eggs in the pan, stirring them as they begin to set, until half cooked, but still runny in places.

Toss over the feta, then place the pan under the grill for 5-6 mins until omelet is puffed up and golden. Cut into wedges and serve straight from the pan. You can refrigerate it and have some the following day.

Prawn and Avocado Cocktail

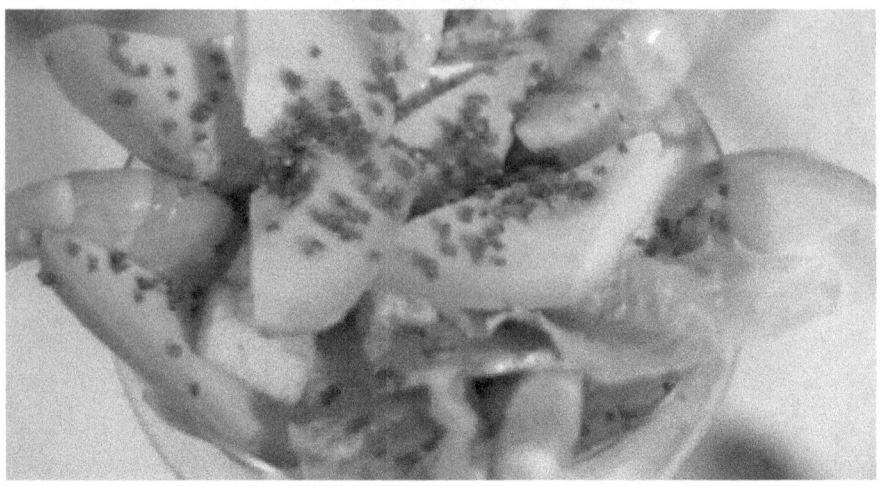

Dressing
juice of ½ lime
juice of ½ orange
segments of the orange
4 tablespoons extra virgin olive o
sea salt and cracked black pepper to season
Salad
1 trimmed fennel bulb cut into small slices
1 destoned avocado thinly sliced
200g cooked king prawns
3 finely chopped spring onions
1 bag washed wild rocket
1 chopped chive

This is a much healthier version of the classic prawn cocktail made with a marie rose sauce or mayonnaise and ketchup.

Make the dressing by mixing the oil and citrus juices together in a small bowl with some salt and pepper, then set aside. In a bowl, toss all the other ingredients, except the rocket, together with the orange segments and half of the dressing. Scatter the rocket leaves into 4 Martini glasses or small bowls, pile the salad into the centre, then drizzle with the remaining dressing just before serving.

Prawn and Chorizo Frittata

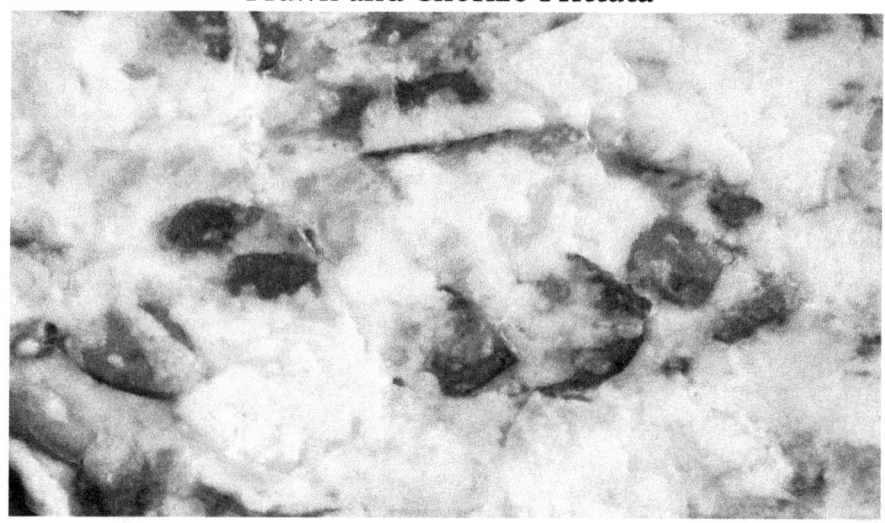

1 medium onion cut into slices
1 clove of garlic finely chopped
1 green pepper cut into small slices
50g chorizo
2 tsp olive oil
knob of butter
5 free range or omega 3 eggs
1 tbsp milk
1 cup of cooked peeled prawns
sea salt and cracked black pepper

Heat grill to medium. In a 20cm frying pan, fry the onion, green pepper, garlic and chorizo in the oil over a low heat. Cook for 4-5 mins, stirring occasionally until the onion is soft. Take the pan off the heat, pour out any excess fat from the chorizo, then stir in the beaten eggs and milk with some seasoning.

Stir in the prawns and return to a low heat for 10-12 mins until all but the very top of the frittata is set. Flash it under the grill until golden. Serve in wedges with a leafy salad.

Chicken Marengo

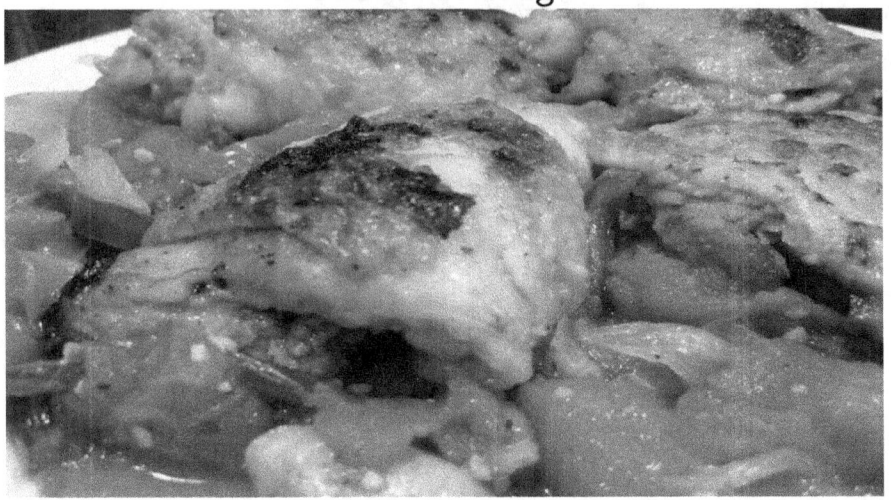

2 tablespoons olive oil
1 cup of button mushroom halved
4 chicken legs with the skin removed
1 can of chopped tomatoes
1 chicken stock cube
½ cup of black olives
1 sliced onion
1 diced garlic clove
handful of chopped flat leaf parsley
sea salt and cracked black pepper

Heat the oil in a large flameproof casserole dish and stir-fry the onions and garlic for two minutes and then add the mushrooms. Add the chicken legs and cook briefly on each side to color them a little. Pour in the tomatoes, crumble in the stock cube and stir in the olives. Season with black pepper, you shouldn't need salt because there will be enough salt in the chorizo. Cover and simmer for 40 mins until the chicken is tender. Sprinkle with parsley. You could serve this with a nice crispy salad.

Grilled Chicken Escalope and Peppers

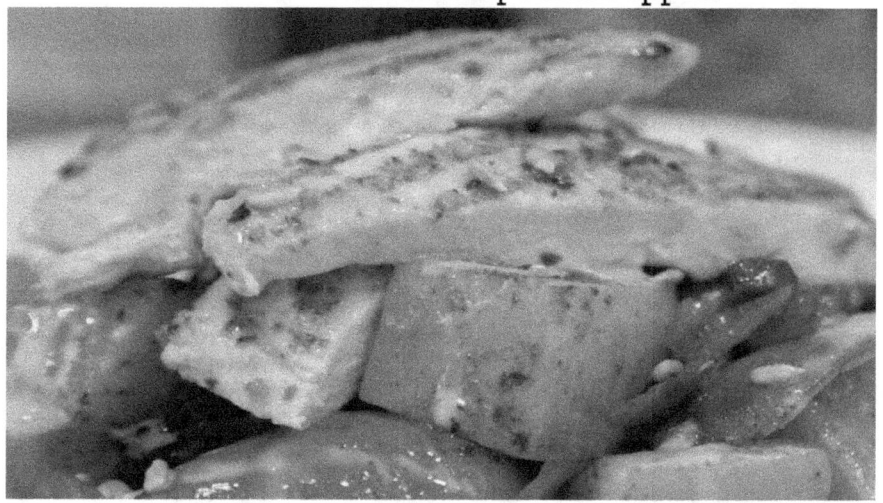

2 chicken breasts
1 sliced yellow pepper
1 sliced red pepper
1 sliced red onion
sea salt and cracked black pepper

Take the chicken breasts, cover them with cling film and beat them down so that are flattened out. Season. Toss the peppers and onion in some olive oil and grill over a high heat until they begin to color. Take out and add the chicken. Grill on both sides. Plate the chicken with the pepper mixture. Season with salt, pepper and olive oil and a little flat leaf parsley.

Grilled Chicken Sprouts and Bacon

2 chicken legs with skin
2 cups of Brussels sprouts, stemmed and chopped
2 tablespoons of coconut oil
2 streaky rashers
1 clove diced garlic
juice of 1 lemon
1/4 cup chicken stock
Pecorino cheese to garnish (optional)

Preheat your oven to 425 degrees. Wash and prep the sprouts. Season chicken with garlic, salt and pepper and grill in a griddle pan with the oil. Leave them be and allow them get crispy. Cut the bacon into pieces and add to the pan until crisp. Add the sprouts. Add a little olive oil if it is too dry. Then add the stock and lemon juice. Bake in the oven for 20-25 minutes until the chicken is fully cooked. Garnish with grated cheese and serve. You can use this recipes for a Paleo diet if you leave out the cheese.

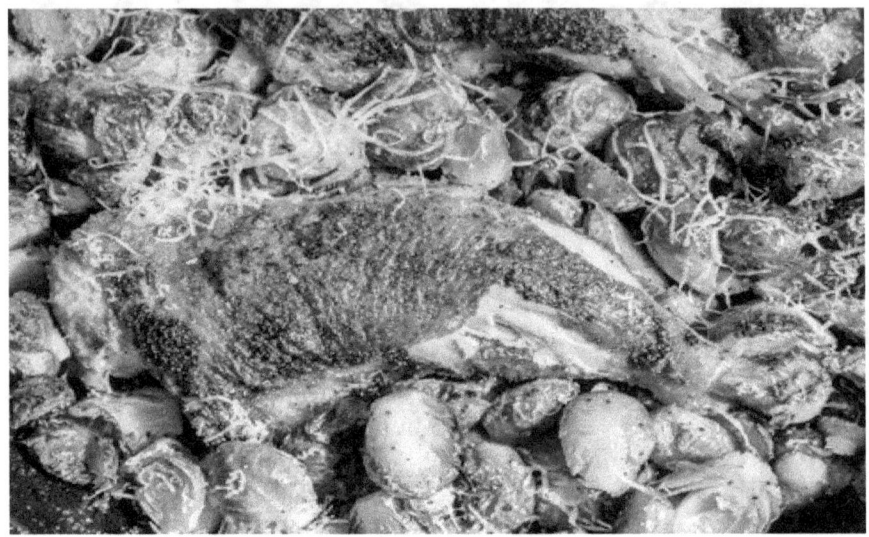

Middle Eastern Shakshuka

¼ cup of extra virgin olive oil
½ diced onion
1 finely chopped garlic clove
1 diced red pepper
clove garlic, minced
1 diced red pepper
2 cups of chopped vine tomatoes
2 tbsp tomato paste
¼ teaspoon of chili flakes
1 tsp chili powder (mild)
1 tsp cumin
1 tsp paprika
5-6 free range or omega 3 eggs
handful of chopped flat leaf parsley

Heat the oil in a pan and cook the onions, garlic and peppers. Add tomatoes and tomato paste to pan, stir till blended. Add spices and allow mixture to simmer over medium heat for 5-7 minutes till it starts to reduce. Season to taste. Crack the eggs directly over the tomato mixture, spacing them so they don't touch. Cover the pan for 10-15 minutes, or until the eggs are cooked and the sauce has slightly reduced. Keep an eye on the skillet to make sure that the sauce doesn't reduce too much, which can lead to burning. Garnish with flat leaf parsley

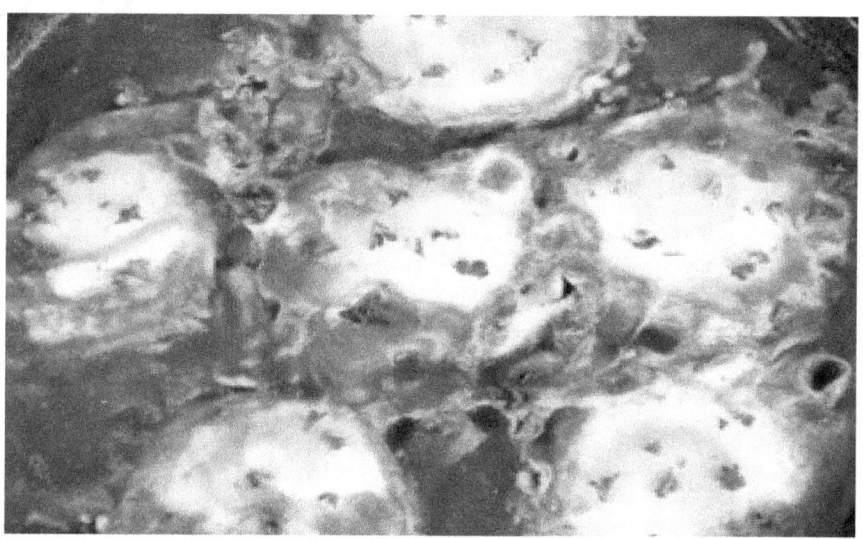

Courgette Spaghetti

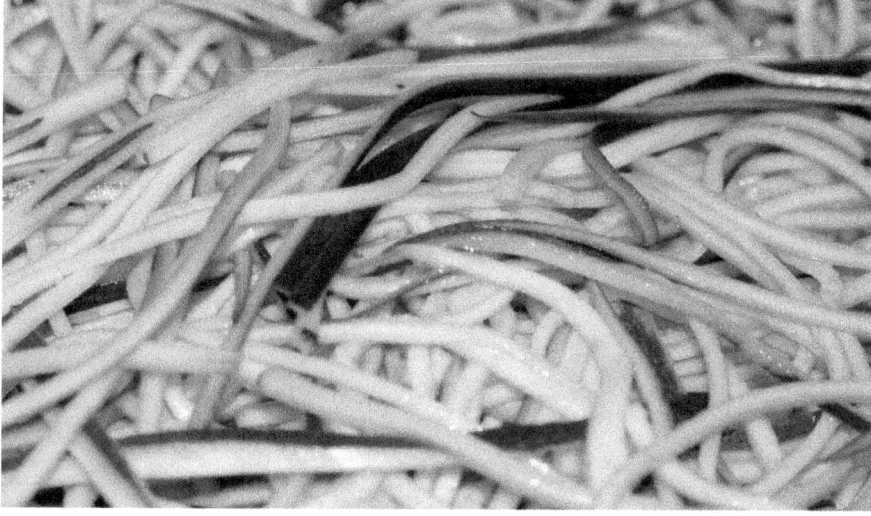

Let me begin by saying that this isn't real spaghetti. It's courgettes or zucchinis as they are called in America finely sliced preferably with a mandolin so they should resemble the above picture.

4 courgettes thinly sliced
1 clove of finely chopped garlic
6 slices streaky bacon
½ cup of chopped scallions
2 cups broccoli florets
½ cup of basil pesto
fresh Parmesan cheese, for garnish
sea salt and cracked black pepper

Place courgette strips in a colander over a bowl or in the sink. Sprinkle with salt and toss to combine. Let them sit for 15 minutes while the salt extracts the moisture. Drain. Meanwhile, cook bacon in a skillet over medium heat until crisp, turning frequently. Allow to cool and then chop into small pieces. Return the pan to the heat with the bacon juices and fry the broccoli onion and garlic. Add the courgettes and pesto. Mix together and serve garnishing with the cheese.

THE GLUTEN FREE DIET

WHAT IS IT?

A gluten-free diet is a diet that excludes the protein gluten. Gluten is the name of a family of proteins present in grains like wheat, spelt, rye and barley and a cross between wheat and rye called triticale. There are two main gluten proteins, called gliadin and glutenin. It is the gliadin part that causes the harmful effects.

When wheat flour is mixed with water, the gluten proteins form a sticky cross-linking network that has a glue-like consistency. The name glu-ten is derived from this glue-like property which makes dough elastic, and gives it the ability to rise during bread making.

The Gluten-free diet is primarily used to treat celiac disease. Gluten causes inflammation in the small intestines of people with celiac disease. Eating a gluten-free diet helps people with celiac disease control these signs and symptoms and prevent complications.

It may interest you to know that a 2013 study showed that a massive 30% of Americans are actively trying to avoid gluten. Although the harmful effects of gluten are controversial among health experts, it is known that several health conditions respond positively to a gluten-free diet.

People who begin a gluten-free diet for the first time may find it frustrating. But if you are patient and creative the chances are that you will find there are many foods that you already eat that are gluten-free. As I already said the gluten-free diet is a treatment for celiac disease but some people who don't have celiac disease also may have symptoms when they eat gluten.

This is called non-celiac gluten sensitivity. People with non-celiac gluten sensitivity may benefit from a gluten-free diet. But people with celiac disease must be gluten-free to prevent symptoms and disease-related complications. Switching to a gluten-free diet is a big step. Some find themselves initially deprived by the diet's restrictions.

But there are more and more gluten free products on our shelves every day. If you can't find them in your area, check with a celiac support group or search online. If you're just starting with a gluten-free diet, it's a good idea to consult a dietitian who can answer your questions and offer advice about how to avoid gluten while still eating a healthy, balanced diet.

WHAT YOU CANNOT EAT
WHEAT
All kinds of wheat, including whole wheat, wheat flour, wheat germ and wheat bran.
SPELT
RYE
BARLEY
EINKORN
TRITICALE
KAMUT.
OTHERS
Durum flour, farina, graham flour, semolina.

The following food usually contain gluten, and should be avoided unless specifically labelled "gluten-free," or made strictly with gluten-free ingredients:
BREAD
Including croutons.
PASTA
CEREALS
BEER
CAKES, PIES, COOKIES, CRACKERS AND PASTRIES
SAUCES
All kinds of sauces especially soy; gravies and dressings.

Remember that gluten can be found in all sorts of processed foods so stick to whole, single ingredient foods as much as possible. Generally speaking, oats do not contain gluten, and are well tolerated in people with celiac disease. However, sometimes oats are processed in the same facilities as wheat, so be careful about cross contamination.

My advice is that unless specifically labelled gluten-free, consider avoiding oats if you have celiac disease. Also keep in mind that certain supplements and medications may contain gluten. The bottom line is that you must always read the labels.

WHAT YOU CAN EAT
Believe it or not there are plenty of healthy and nutritious foods that are naturally gluten free. Here are some examples of the most common types:
MEAT
Chicken, turkey, lamb, beef, and pork.
FISH
Salmon, trout, haddock and prawns.
EGGS
All kinds but free range, pastured and Omega-3 enriched eggs are best.
DAIRY
Milk, cheese, and yogurt.
VEGETABLES
Broccoli, kale, Brussels sprouts, carrots, peppers and onions.
FRUIT
Apples, avocados, bananas, oranges, pears, strawberries, and blueberries.
LEGUMES
Lentils, beans, and peanuts.
NUTS
Almonds, walnuts, and macadamia nuts.
TUBERS
Potatoes, and sweet potatoes. But not French fries.
HEALTHY FATS
Olive oil, avocado oil, butter, and coconut oil.
HERBS AND SPICES
GLUTEN FREE GRAINS
Quinoa, rice, corn, flax, millet, sorghum, tapioca, buckwheat, arrowroot, amaranth, as well as oats (if labelled gluten-free).
OTHERS
Dark chocolate.

WHAT TO DRINK
You can drink water, coffee and tea on a gluten-free diet. You can even drink fruit juices and sugary drinks but remember they are high in sugar. As regards alcohol, beer should be avoided unless labelled gluten-free, but most wines and spirits don't contain gluten.

SIMPLE MEAL PLANNERS BUT ALSO CHECK THE RECIPES
As with the previous three diets I am going to give you set daily meal plans

for six mini meals. Again, the planner is a template, switch it around to suit yourself. And don't forget to try some of the delicious recipes.

	SUNDAY
BREAKFAST	Scrambled Eggs with Vegetables
ELEVEN	Bowl of Berries
LUNCH	Beef Stir Fry with Red and Green Peppers
AFTERNOON	Bowl of Nuts
DINNER	Chicken Salad
NIGHT-TIME	Banana
TREATS	Either glass of Wine or two squares of Chocolate (70%)

	MONDAY
BREAKFAST	Gluten Free Oats with Whole Milk
ELEVEN	Bowl of Raisins
LUNCH	Smoothie with Coconut Milk, Chocolate Whey Protein powder, Berries and Almonds
AFTERNOON	Apple
DINNER	Salmon fried in Butter with a Side Salad
NIGHT-TIME	Banana
TREATS	Either glass of Wine or two squares of Chocolate (70%)

	TUESDAY
BREAKFAST	Omelette with Red Pepper fried in Butter
ELEVEN	Apple
LUNCH	Tuna Salad dressed in Olive Oil
AFTERNOON	Bowl of Nuts
DINNER	Burger without Bun served with Potatoes fried in Butter
NIGHT-TIME	Banana
TREATS	Either glass of Wine or two squares of Chocolate (70%)

	WEDNESDAY
BREAKFAST	Greek Yoghurt with Sliced Fruit
ELEVEN	Bowl of Nuts
LUNCH	Grilled Chicken with Salsa
AFTERNOON	Apple
DINNER	Meatballs with Vegetables and Brown Rice
NIGHT-TIME	Banana
TREATS	Either glass of Wine or two squares of Chocolate (70%)

	THURSDAY
BREAKFAST	Fried Eggs and Peppers fried in Coconut Oil
ELEVEN	Apple
LUNCH	Tuna Salad
AFTERNOON	Smoothie
DINNER	Striploin Steak with Vegetables
NIGHT-TIME	Banana
TREATS	Either glass of Wine or two squares of Chocolate (70%)

	FRIDAY
BREAKFAST	Oatmeal with Whole Milk
ELEVEN	Bowl of Nuts
LUNCH	Beef Burger without Bun and served with a Salsa
AFTERNOON	Apple
DINNER	Baked Salmon with Vegetables
NIGHT-TIME	Banana
TREATS	Either glass of Wine or two squares of Chocolate (70%)

	SATURDAY
BREAKFAST	Bacon and Eggs fried in Butter
ELEVEN	Organic Yogurt with Berries
LUNCH	Tuna with Salsa
AFTERNOON	Low Carb Smoothie (Coconut Milk, Berries, Almonds and Protein powder)
DINNER	Grilled Chicken Wings with Vegetables and Sweet Potato
NIGHT-TIME	Bowl of Cherries
TREATS	Either glass of Wine or two squares of Chocolate (70%)

15 GLUTEN FREE DIET RECIPES

Potato Frittata

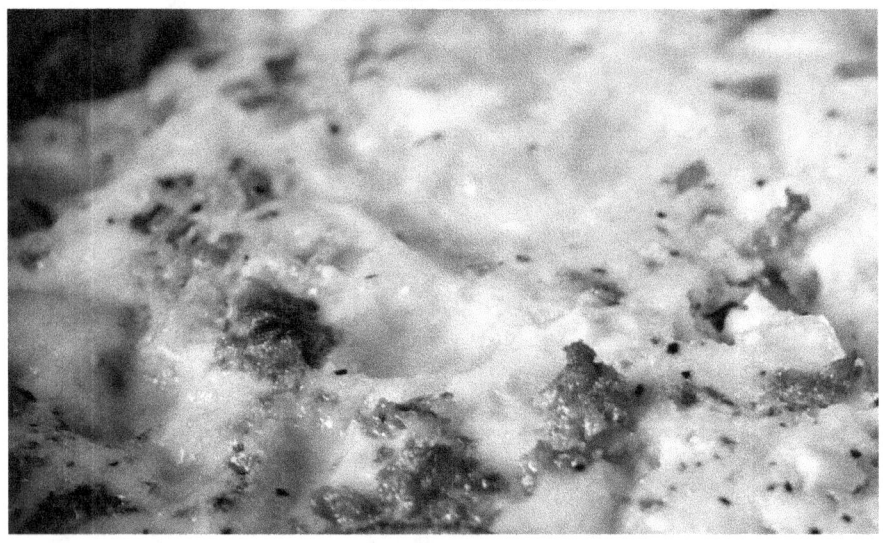

1 large baking potato
5 organic, free range, pastured or omega 3 eggs
Handful of chopped leaf parsley
2 tablespoons olive oil
1 small chopped onion
½ chopped red pepper
½ cup chopped button mushrooms
1 clove finely chopped garlic
½ cup of chopped ham

1 sliced tomato
¼ cup of shredded cheddar cheese
sea salt and cracked black pepper

Chop the potato into cubes and boil until just cooked. Set aside. Fry the mushrooms until cooked. Add in the beaten eggs, parsley and ham. Season and sprinkle the cheese on top and bake in the oven until firm and cooked.

Parma Wrapped Prawns

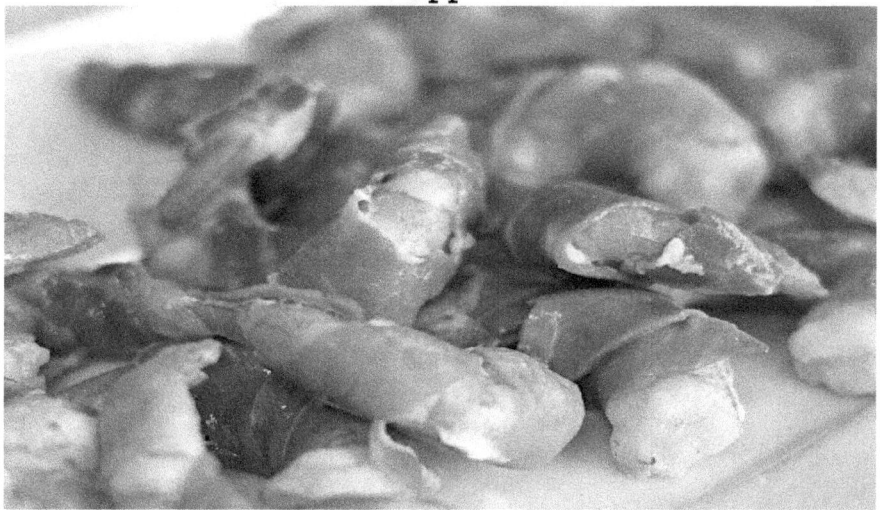

10 large frozen peeled deveined shrimp, thawed
1 tablespoon chopped fresh basil
2 tablespoons extra-virgin olive oil
½ teaspoon lemon zest
5 thin slices Parma ham
cooking spray
sea salt and cracked black pepper
8 lemon wedges, for serving

In a bowl mix prawns, basil, olive oil, lemon zest, salt and pepper. Set aside. Cut the Parma into strips and wrap around each prawn leaving the tail exposed. Spray with the oil and flash griddle in the pan until cooked. Serve immediately with with lemon wedges.

Alternatively, you can buy the prawns already cooked. Marinate with the olive oil, zest and basil and cover with Parma ham and serve with lemon.

Three Apple Chicken Salad

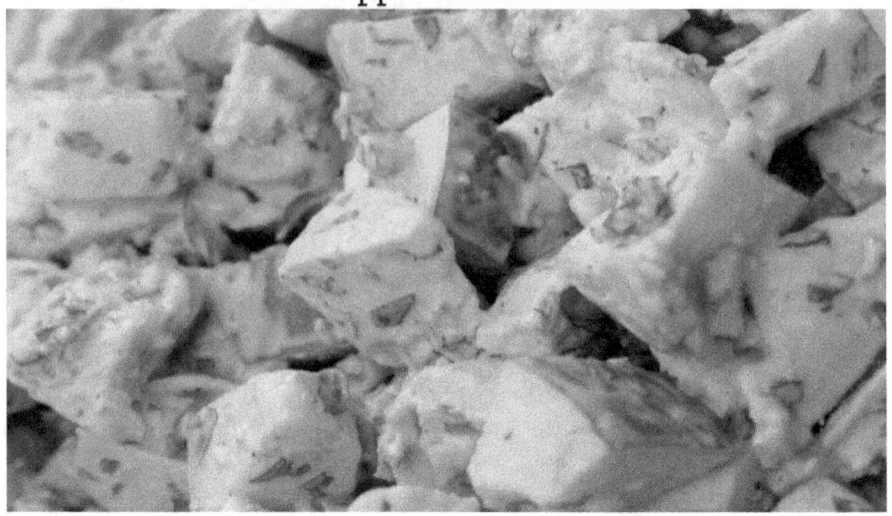

2 diced cooked chicken breasts
1 diced green apple
1 diced red apple
1 diced Granny Smith
½ cup of diced celery
3 tablespoons chopped pecans, toasted
¼ cup of yogurt
2 tablespoons reduced-fat sour cream
1 teaspoons stone-ground mustard
1 teaspoon dried tarragon
juice of ¼ orange
sea salt and cracked black pepper

Mix chicken, apples, celery, juice and pecans in bowl and season. Combine the yogurt, sour cream, mustard, and tarragon. Pour dressing over chicken mixture; toss gently to coat. Cover; chill at least 30 minutes

Chicken White Bean and Spinach Soup
2 tablespoon olive oil
1 chopped onion
2 cloves finely chopped garlic
1 tablespoon chopped fresh thyme
2 cans cannellini beans rinsed and drained
¼ cup water mixed with ¼ cup white wine
4 diced plum tomatoes

2 cups of chicken broth
3 cups of baby spinach leaves
2 chopped cooked chicken breasts
sea salt and cracked black pepper to season

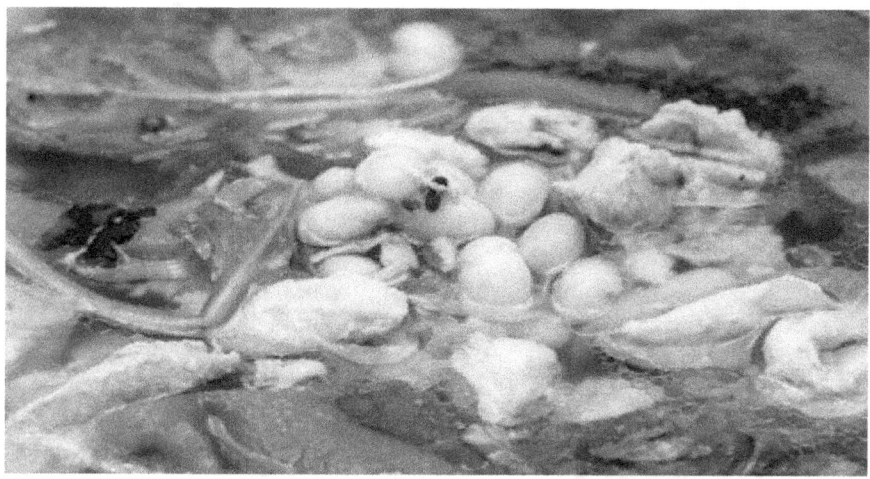

Heat oil in saucepan and add the onion, garlic and thyme. Cook for 3 minutes and add the beans, water, wine, tomatoes, and broth. Increase heat to high until stew begins to bubble. Reduce heat; let simmer for 5 minutes. Add more water, if needed. Drop in the spinach and chicken. Cook until the chicken is hot. Season, bowl and serve.

Poached Cod with Pesto and Green Beans

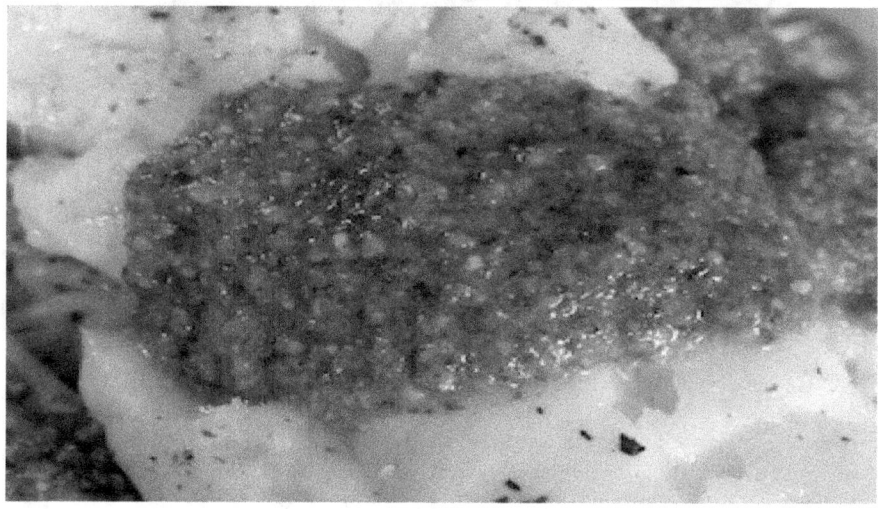

2 tablespoon extra-virgin olive oil
1 pound green beans
1 finely chopped onion
2 cod pieces
1 cup chicken broth
½ cup of pesto
sea salt and cracked black pepper
lemon wedges for serving

Heat oil in a large pan and add the beans and onion for about two minutes. Season the cod and spread the beans into a flat layer in the pan and gently place the cod on top. Increase heat to high, add broth, cover and cook until the fish is just cooked through, 4 to 6 minutes. Take out the cod and beans when cooked. Leave the broth, turn up the heat and reduce by half. Pour the sauce over the fish and beans, top the fish with the pesto and serve with lemon wedges.

Lemon and Lime Grilled Chicken Thighs

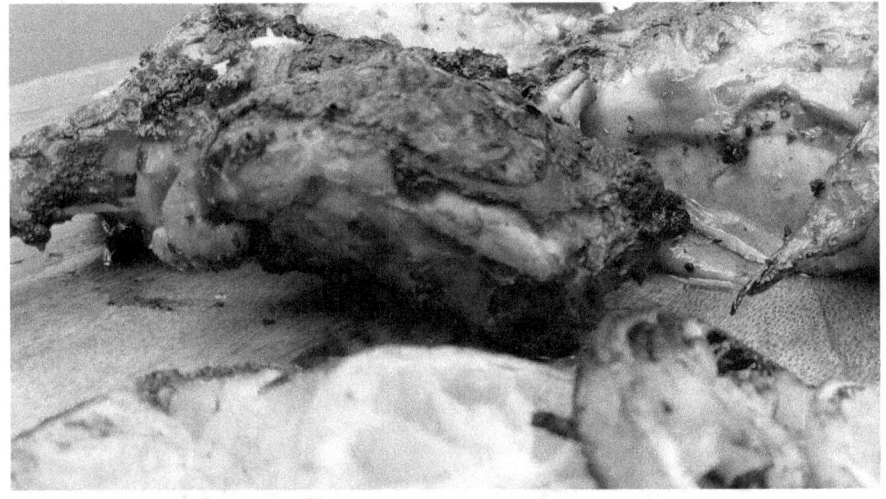

4 large chicken thighs with skin removed
1 finely chopped shallot
2 tablespoons finely chopped fresh ginger
2 tablespoons canola oil
½ tablespoon lime zest
½ tablespoon of lemon zest
1 tablespoons lime juice
1 tablespoon of lemon juice
1 teaspoon ground cinnamon

½ teaspoon freshly grated nutmeg
pinch of cayenne pepper
sea salt and cracked black pepper to season

Line a baking sheet with foil and coat with cooking spray. Place the chicken on it. Mix shallots, ginger, oil, lemon and lime zest and juice, cinnamon, salt, pepper, nutmeg and cayenne and rub into the chicken. Cover and refrigerate for at least 2 hours but preferably overnight. Preheat the griddle to high. Grill the chicken until cooked on all sides. Serve with a salsa.

Red Cabbage Salad

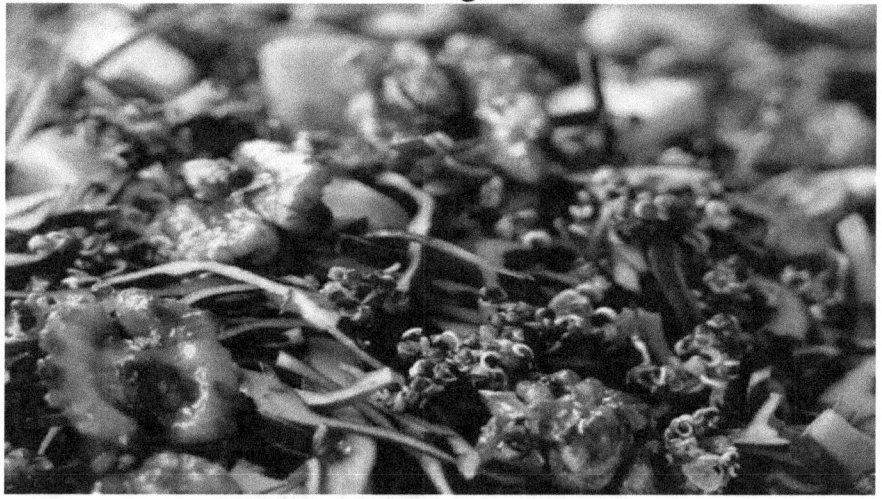

Vinaigrette
1 tablespoon crumbled blue cheese
¼ cup extra-virgin olive oil
3 tablespoons red-wine vinegar
1 tablespoon Dijon mustard
sea salt and cracked black pepper to season
Salad
1 tablespoon extra-virgin olive oil
1 teaspoon butter
1 cup walnuts
3 tablespoons pure maple syrup
8 cups very thinly sliced red cabbage
2 scallions, thinly sliced
¼ cup crumbled blue cheese (optional)

To prepare vinaigrette mix 1 tablespoon blue cheese, 1/4 cup oil, vinegar, mustard, salt and pepper in a mini food processor or blender; process until creamy. To make the salad first cook the walnuts in butter. Season. Set aside. Place cabbage and scallions in a large bowl. Toss with the vinaigrette. Serve topped with blue cheese and the walnuts.

Roasted Baby Potatoes and Sweet Onion

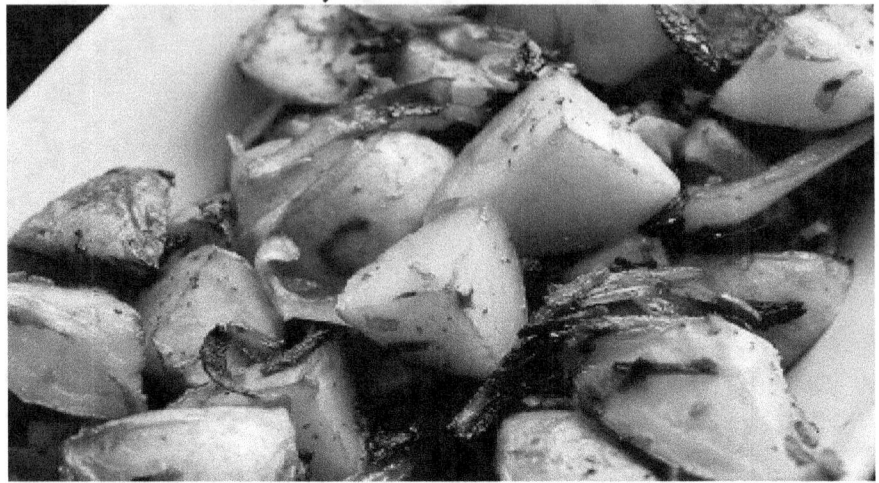

2 pounds Yukon Gold potatoes, scrubbed, cut into 1-inch-thick wedges
5 tablespoons extra-virgin olive oil
2 medium sweet onions cut into 1-inch-thick wedges with root ends intact
1 tablespoon chopped fresh rosemary
Sea salt and cracked black pepper

Preheat oven. Boil the potatoes until almost tender. Drain and return to the pot. Divide 3 tablespoons oil between 2 baking sheets, tilting to coat. Place the pans in the oven to heat for 5 minutes. When the potatoes are dry, drizzle with the remaining 2 tablespoons oil. Season.

Gently toss until coated. Add onions and gently turn with your hands to coat, trying not to break them up. Arrange the potatoes and onions, cut side down, on the hot baking sheets. Roast until browned and crisp on the bottom. Remove and sprinkle with rosemary. Season.

Baked Sea Bass with Lemon Caper Dressing

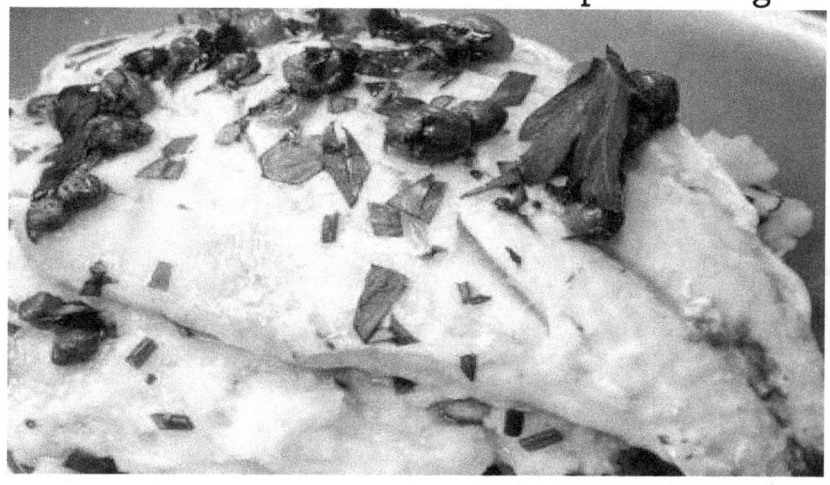

4 sea bass fillets
2 tablespoons olive oil
Dressing
3 tbsp extra virgin olive oil
grated zest 1 lemon
2 tbsp lemon juice
2 tbsp small capers
2 tsp gluten-free Dijon mustard
handful of chopped flat-leaf parsley
sea salt and cracked black pepper

To make the dressing, mix the oil with the lemon zest and juice, capers, mustard, some seasoning and 1 tbsp water. Heat the oven to 220C/200C fan/gas 7. Line a baking tray with baking parchment and put the fish, skin-side up, on top. Brush the skin with oil and season.

Bake for 7 mins or until the flesh flakes when tested with a knife. Arrange the fish on warm serving plates, spoon over the dressing and sprinkle with parsley leaves. Serve on a bed of buttered mash.

Spanish Meatballs and Bean Stew

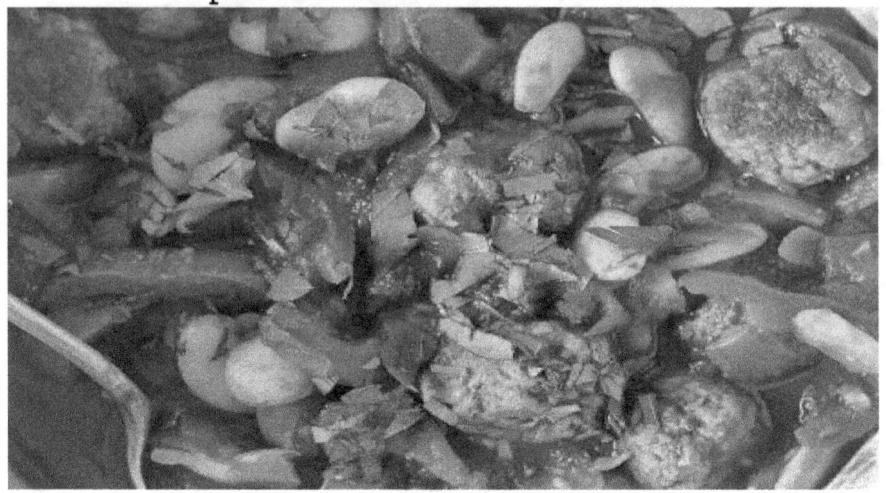

This recipe is courtesy of the BBC.
350g lean pork mince
2 tsp olive oil
1 large red onion, chopped
2 sliced red peppers
3 garlic cloves, crushed
1 tbsp sweet smoked paprika
2 cans chopped tomatoes
400g can butter beans, drained
2 tsp golden caster sugar
handful of flat leaf parsley

Season the pork and shape into small meatballs. Heat the oil in a large pan, add the meatballs and cook for 5 mins. Put aside. Add the onion and peppers to the pan and cook for a further 5 minutes. Stir in the garlic and paprika. Then add the tomatoes. Cover with a lid and simmer for 10 mins. Uncover, stir in the beans, the sugar and some seasoning, then simmer for a further 10 mins, uncovered. Just before serving, stir in the parsley.

Gluten Free Oatmeal and Berries
1 cup whole milk
1 cup water
½ teaspoon kosher salt
1 teaspoon vanilla extract
1 cup whole rolled gluten-free oats
cup of mixed berries

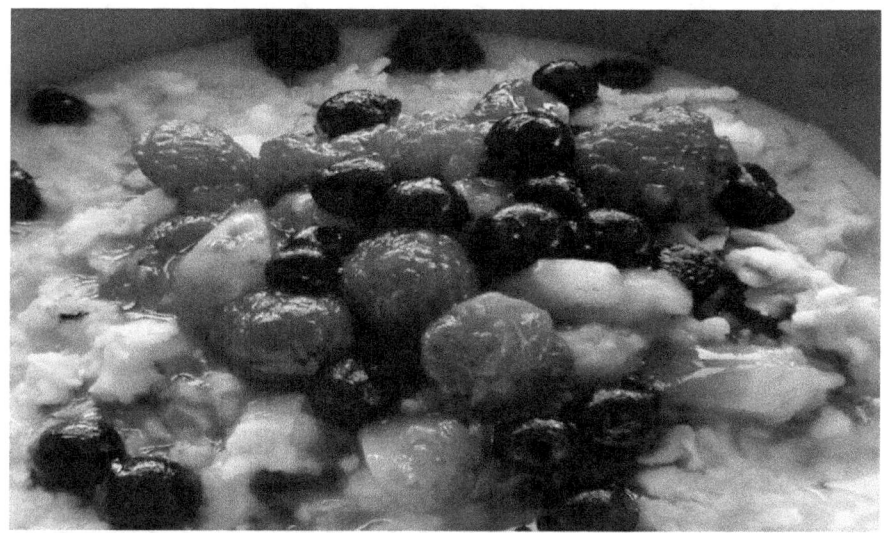

Pour the milk and water into a saucepan over a medium heat. Add the salt and vanilla extract. Bring the liquids to a boil. When the milky water is boiling, pour in the oats. Stir vigorously. When the water returns to a boil, turn down the heat to low. Simmer the oats, stirring every few minutes, until the oats are creamy and plump, the liquid fully absorbed, about 15 minutes. Turn off the heat and cover the pan. Let the oatmeal sit for five minutes to fully absorb the liquid. Top with berries and serve.

Roasted Cauliflower

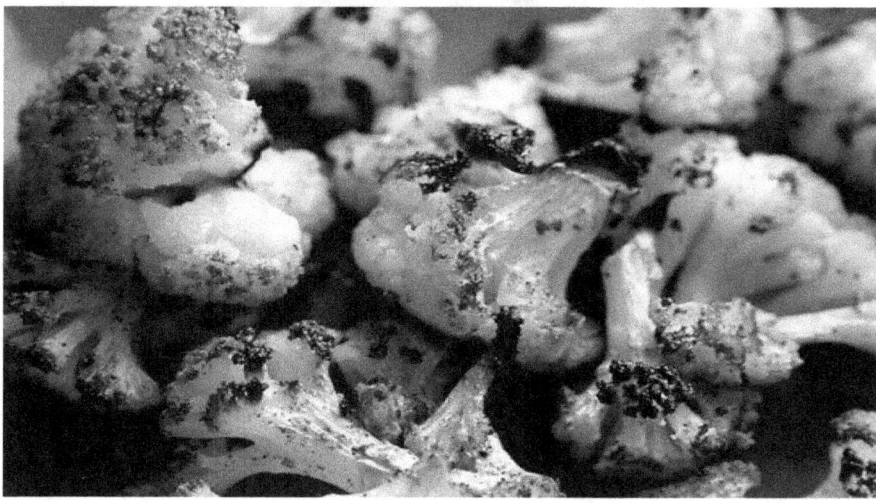

1 head cauliflower (about 2 pounds), cut into small florets
2 tablespoons extra-virgin olive oil
6 cloves chopped garlic
pinch of cayenne pepper
2 teaspoons roughly chopped fresh thyme leaves
sea salt and cracked black pepper to season

Preheat the oven to 450 degrees F. Toss the cauliflower with the olive oil, and garlic on a baking sheet; sprinkle with the salt, pepper and thyme and toss again. Roast until golden and tender, about 20 minutes. Transfer to a serving bowl and serve

Roasted Sweet Potato with Honey

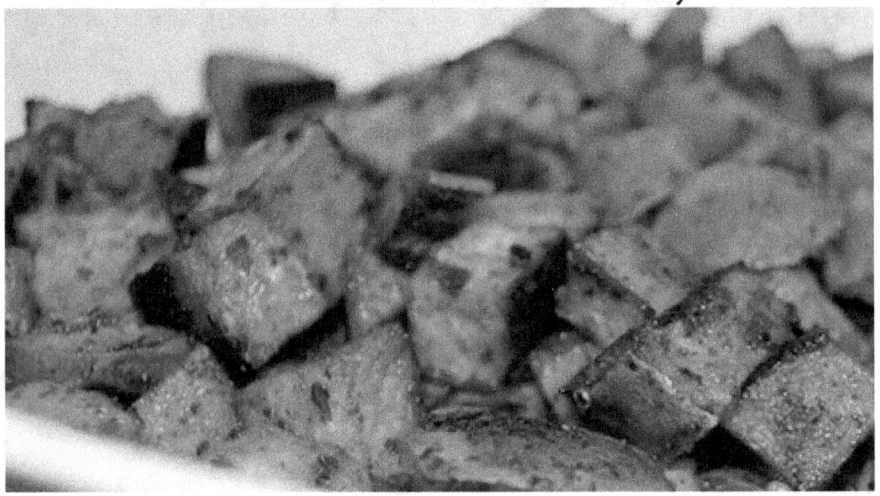

4 sweet potatoes, peeled and cut into 1-inch cubes
½ cup extra-virgin olive oil
3 tablespoons honey
2 teaspoons ground cinnamon
sea salt and cracked black pepper

Preheat oven to 375 degrees F. Place the potatoes on a roasting tray. Drizzle the oil, honey, cinnamon, salt and pepper over the potatoes. Roast for 25 to 30 minutes in oven or until tender.

Indian Spiced Salmon

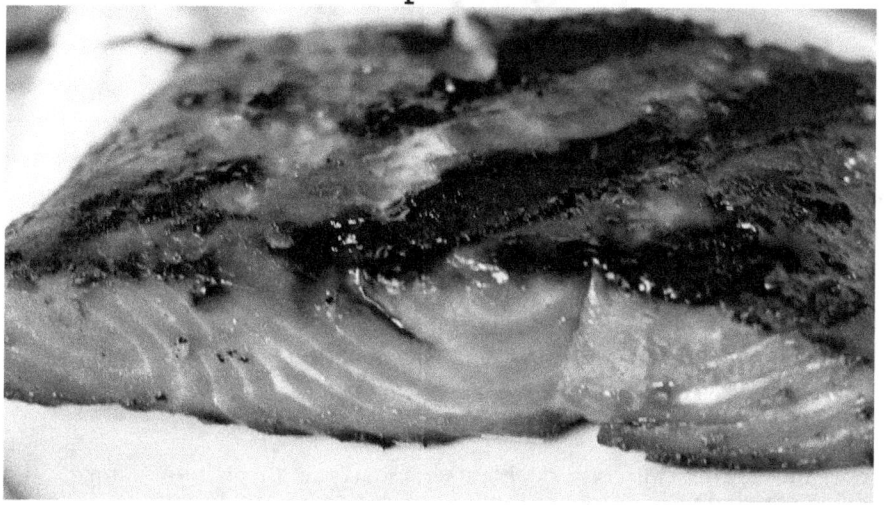

½ teaspoon ground ginger
½ teaspoon garam masala
½ teaspoon ground coriander
½ teaspoon ground turmeric
1 tablespoon honey
pinch of salt
pinch of ground red pepper
4 skinless salmon fillets
cooking spray

Combine first 6 ingredients. Rub spice mixture evenly over fillets. Place fillets on a pan with cooking spray. Cover with foil; broil 7 minutes. Remove foil; grill an additional 4 minutes. Serve with a salsa.

Gluten Free Crab Cakes

14 vegetable gluten free crackers
½ cup mayonnaise
3 tablespoons finely minced celery
2 tablespoons minced fresh parsley
1 ½ teaspoons seafood seasoning
1 teaspoon dry mustard
1 tablespoon lemon juice
2 large eggs
1 lb lump crabmeat
gluten free all-purpose flour mix
Olive oil

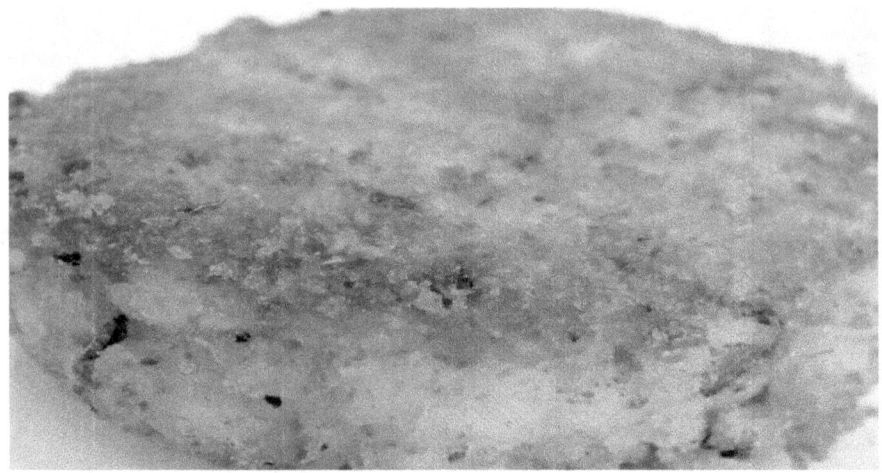

Put the crackers into a food blender and blend them into crumbs. In a mixing bowl, blend together mayonnaise, celery, parsley, seafood seasoning, dry mustard, lemon juice and eggs. Gently stir in the crabmeat. Line surface with flour mix. Form mixture into 6 cakes carefully, pressing just firmly enough to shape. Let sit for 5 minutes. Coat a large pan with olive oil and set it over medium heat. Once it is hot, add the crab cakes and cook until browned. Turn carefully and cook the second sides.

Grilled Pork Loin

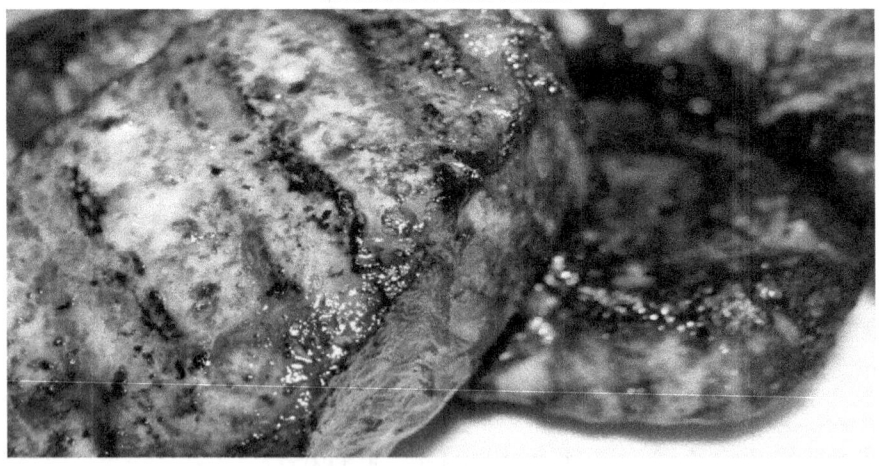

4 chopped garlic cloves
4 teaspoons chopped fresh rosemary
4 pork loin chops
sea salt and cracked black pepper

Preheat oven to 400°. Line a roasting pan with foil. Mix first 4 ingredients in bowl. Rub garlic mixture over pork. Place pork, fat side down, in prepared roasting pan; cook 30 minutes. urn roast fat side up; continue cooking for about 20-25 minutes. Remove from oven; let stand 10 minutes. Serve with a salsa.

ABOUT THE AUTHOR

David Elio Malocco studied law at University College Dublin, Ireland; psychology at the Open University in Milton Keynes, England; Film Studies at New York University; and Creative Writing at Oxford University England.

He has written and directed three feature films, three documentaries and seven shorts and has written twenty books on such diverse topics as criminal profiling, crime scene analysis, psychotherapy, psychology, the Beatles conspiracy, serial killers, anthropophagy, cooking and now nutrition.

His book *How to Commit the Perfect Murder* has been on the Amazon best seller's list for two years.

He is founder of the charity We Will Work it Out which specializes in mental health care for young people. He lives in Ireland with his wife and three rescue dogs.

www.ingramcontent.com/pod-product-compliance
Lightning Source LLC
Chambersburg PA
CBHW071152290526
45788CB00001BA/439